S0-EKK-343

THE
MENTZER METHOD
TO FITNESS

Mark T. Summersen

7/7/80

THE MENTZER METHOD TO FITNESS

A Revolutionary Weight-Training System for Men and Women

Mike Mentzer
with Ardy Friedberg

WILLIAM MORROW AND COMPANY, INC.
New York   1980

Copyright © 1980 by Mike Mentzer and Ardy Friedberg

All rights reserved. No part of this book may be reproduced or utilized in any form or by any means, electronic or mechanical, including photocopying, recording or by any information storage and retrieval system, without permission in writing from the Publisher. Inquiries should be addressed to William Morrow and Company, Inc., 105 Madison Ave., New York, N. Y. 10016.

Library of Congress Cataloging in Publication Data

Mentzer, Mike.
    The Mentzer method to fitness.

    "Morrow quill paperbacks."
    Includes index.
    1. Bodybuilding.   2. Physical fitness.
3. Nutrition.   I. Friedberg, Ardy, joint author.
II. Title.
GV546.5.M46   1980b   646.7′5   79-27849
ISBN 0-688-03636-8
ISBN 0-688-08636-5 pbk.

Printed in the United States of America

First Morrow Quill Paperback Edition

1   2   3   4   5   6   7   8   9   10

In memory of my mother,
Marie Mentzer, whose loving
care and nurturance, when
it really counted, made
this book possible.

—M.M.

———————

For Susie:
I couldn't have done it
without her.

—A.F.

Contents

THE
MENTZER METHOD
TO FITNESS

PART I

Chapter 1

Mr. Universe—The Mentzer
Method Proves Itself

It's November 20, 1978. The setting is the lavish Centro de Convenciones Acapulco. Oscar State, secretary of the Judging Committee of the International Federation of Bodybuilders, is at the microphone.

The enthusiastic and noisy crowd has finally quieted down in anticipation of State's announcement. There is tension in the air and I'm aware of a tingling sensation all over my body. The moment everyone has been waiting for is here.

"Ladies and gentlemen. The winner, with a perfect score of 300 points, the first perfect score ever awarded in the history of international bodybuilding competition, the new Mr. Universe, Mike Mentzer of the United States!"

Pandemonium. I am a jumble of sensations. I feel a tremendous surge of great strength and at the same time a little light-headed. I hear the crowd of 2,700 erupt in cheers and the chant of "Ment-zer, Ment-zer" as it builds in the back of the auditorium and breaks like a wave toward the stage. After all the years of work, the discipline, the sweat, I've reached the top of the amateur bodybuilding world.

In the flurry of back slapping and hand shaking that followed the announcement of my victory over ninety of the greatest bodybuilders in the world, I bounced around in a happy daze, somewhat disoriented, not yet realizing I had just fulfilled a lifetime

13

dream. Winning the Mr. America title had been very exciting but nothing like this.

It wasn't until several hours later, after I had had some time to reflect on the events of the day, all the planning and all the training that led up to this moment, that the full significance of what had happened, the reality of my triumph began to register. Not only had I won the Mr. Universe title, the most prestigious crown in all of amateur bodybuilding, but I had received a perfect score as well. Even the great Arnold Schwarzenegger never received a perfect score in international competition.

But equally as important as the victory, the title, and the perfect score was the deep sense of satisfaction that I felt because the Mr. Universe title finally gave credibility to my radically new and highly controversial training and dieting philosophy, a philosophy that stresses short, high-intensity workouts coupled with a sensible, well-balanced diet.

I know that every one of the other contestants in the Mr. Universe contest that year trained six days a week, at least two hours a day, and that many of them trained four hours a day. That's twenty-four hours a week, the equivalent of three full work days.

In sharp contrast, my training sessions then (and now) rarely exceeded thirty minutes, three times a week—a grand total of less than two hours a week in the gym, roughly one tenth as long as my competitors. Not only that, but during those long arduous hours spent in the gym, they made their task all the more torturous because their extremely low-carbohydrate, high-protein diets were depriving their bodies of a sorely needed energy source. I know bodybuilders who cut their carbohydrate intake to nearly zero during contest training. This is sheer madness since the body's primary fuel comes from carbohydrate and fat, not from protein which isn't used as fuel to any appreciable extent as long as the body's energy supplies are adequate.

My precompetition diet, on the other hand, consists almost entirely of tasty, satisfying, energy-producing carbohydrates. For example, before a contest, my typical breakfast usually includes juice, eggs, potatoes, toast, and coffee with cream, and it is a rare day that I don't indulge in my favorite food—ice cream. It's important to note, though, that I don't follow this diet recklessly. During training I'm burning a tremendous number of calories and the kind of breakfast I described barely replaces the energy consumed during my high-intensity sessions.

I am well aware that my workout routine and my diet both fly in the face of decades of conventional bodybuilding "wisdom" and that even the whisper of my name is heresy in some gyms. But after Acapulco, I can't help but think that now, even the most skeptical of my critics will have to take a closer look at my approach and will have to concede, however grudgingly, that I am right—that thirty minutes of intense work, three times a week, a total of an hour and a half, is more productive than twenty-four hours of tedious labor.

But whether or not the serious bodybuilders give credence to my training methods, the most exciting aspect of this new approach to physical and mental well-being is its complete applicability to the beginner, to men and women, to teenagers, and to people past forty. I am thoroughly convinced—and I'm backed up by many exercise physiologists, heart specialists, nutritionists, and psychologists—that what I now call the "Mentzer Method" can be used by anyone and that the benefits—1) greater strength and physical endurance; 2) a more beautiful and well-developed body; 3) greater cardiovascular efficiency; and 4) the relief of physical and mental stress—can be derived by exercising less than two hours a week. The Mentzer Method isn't magic, nothing is. It requires hard work and commitment. But I promise you, the rewards are great.

Chapter 2

The Rise of Weight Training

I first got interested in bodybuilding at the rather tender age of twelve. I clearly remember picking up a copy of one of the popular muscle magazines at the corner drug store, leafing through it, and almost immediately realizing that someday I wanted to look like those massive bodybuilders. This was about the same time most of my friends began thinking seriously about baseball, basketball, football, tennis, and the other, more conventional, sports. In fact, my high school football coach couldn't comprehend my reasons for shunning the glories of the gridiron for the obscurity of the weight room.

Neither could my parents for that matter. They were very concerned because they believed the myths and misconceptions that did, and still do, surround the sport of bodybuilding. After all, they said, what did I really know about the dangers of becoming muscle-bound, about large muscles eventually turning to fat, about the lurking spectre of homosexuality inherent in paying too much attention to my own body. I didn't know any of the answers to the questions that worried them, nor was I terribly concerned.

Looking back, I know now that I was an impressionable, idealistic adolescent whose love affair with bodybuilding was a rather naive romance. Every waking moment during that halcyon period was filled with visions of some far-off day when I too would possess the Herculean physique of my heroes. Glorious images danced through the fog of my adolescent mind. I didn't know about muscle-bound, about fat. I didn't even know what a homosexual was at that time, and I didn't care.

What I did know, and knew it with a passion uncommon to me, was that I wanted to look like the men in the muscle magazines.

Like most young obsessives, I responded to the disapproval of my friends and relatives by withdrawing into the insulated world of the gym. I pursued my goal on my own and for years I continued despite their scorn because I was striving for a noble goal—perfection of the human form. It wasn't until many years later that I realized their disapproval was more historic than experiential, rooted in sociological dogma, man's age-old vacillation about the body, an attitude that has swung from the Greek ideal of a healthy mind in a healthy body to the Victorian rejection of the body and its needs.

Happily, we seem now to be on the upswing of the pendulum where health, beauty, vitality, and fitness are again good and positive virtues. Smoking is out. Exercise and dieting are in. There has been a revolution in men's and women's clothes, a movement toward color and cut that accentuates the body rather than hiding it. The resurrection of the well-muscled, resourceful physical hero—Superman, Wonder Woman, the Incredible Hulk—indicates that the body (the highly developed body at that) has once again assumed its rightful place in the sun.

It's no surprise to me, though it is to some, that weight training has also come to the fore as a physical conditioner. Top professional athletes in every sport are using weights to build strength and endurance. Even joggers, that scantily clad army of fanatics, are turning to weight training to build upper-body strength and flesh out their wraithlike figures.

You don't have to have a crystal ball to see that a move toward bodybuilding is at hand. Weight training could be the fitness mode of the 80s.

Gyms, fitness centers, health spas, and Nautilus training centers are popping up like dandelions on a spring lawn. The health-food industry is booming and nutrition is on everyone's mind. Add to this the large audiences, both live and television, for the Mr. America and Mr. Olympia shows, the big, ecstatic crowds drawn by the lesser known physique shows and local contests around the country, the mass readership of the various muscle magazines, and the estimated 4.7 million current weight trainers (the figure could easily be twice as high), and you have the framework to support a fitness movement that is much more than a fad.

But I have a feeling there is more at work here than a simple desire for physical fitness, as positive as that goal may be. Basic changes in society may be the deeper, though less tangible, reasons for this attention to physical appearance.

The easing of rigid role distinctions between male and female resulting from many kinds of consciousness-raising efforts has awakened all of us. Men are beginning to realize that they have bodies that need to be tended. The assumption of new roles by women has also resulted in a shift in their attitude toward their bodies. Women and girls are exerting themselves physically in organized athletics of all kinds, right alongside men and boys. This is a radical departure for American society, a departure that is challenging traditional lifestyles and values. These new lifestyles and values include a freedom to participate and a desire for beauty and health.

I'm well aware that there are a number of ways of achieving physical fitness. Jogging, the most recent fad to sweep the nation, is one way. The other active sports—tennis, racquetball, swimming, squash—all produce certain beneficial, though limited, results. But none of these sports works on the whole body and the mind as does weight training.

I'm going to say flatly that weight training, using the Mentzer Method, is the best means of achieving a better looking body, building strength, endurance, and vitality, increasing cardiovascular efficiency, and lowering the level of mental stress. Weight training is the only type of exercise capable of delivering all of these benefits in a safe and predictable fashion.

I want to pass on the Mentzer Method, not so you can become a professional and competitive bodybuilder (few people want to and fewer are genetically structured for it), but to help you achieve the state of well-being weight training the Mentzer Method way can provide.

Chapter 3

The Long Road of Discovery

As is the case with most discoveries I arrived at the Mentzer Method through trial and error. I made many mistakes in my quest for the perfect physique, mistakes that held me back, but they were mistakes that taught me a great deal about physical fitness, how to attain it, and how to keep it. This book will help you avoid making the same errors I made.

When I first began training with weights nearly sixteen years ago, I was so enthusiastic and so anxious to look like my hero Bill Pearl (who, by the way, is still in competitive shape at the age of fifty), I was willing to do literally anything necessary to achieve my goal. If someone had told me that working out fourteen hours every day with railroad ties would produce the results I wanted, I would not have bothered to ask how, but headed straight for the nearest railroad yard. That was the nature of my enthusiasm . . . and my ignorance.

When I started training at twelve, and for the first three years after that, I actually trained in a relatively sensible and productive way, thanks to the wisdom of the people who put together the little booklet that came with my first set of weights. It suggested that beginners work out no more than three days a week, performing three sets of exercises for each body part. This amounted to a couple of hours for each workout.

In those three years, with some credit to postpubescent development, I made the best progress of my life. I went from a ninety-five-pound kid (not quite the proverbial ninety-seven-pound weakling) with nine-inch arms to a 165-pound man with 15½-inch arms.

At fifteen I really began to take on the thick, rounded, muscular look of a bodybuilder. It seems strange and funny now, but I remember doing my sets in the backyard on hot summer days and immediately running inside to look in the mirror and admire my arms while they were still pumped up. It was just about then that I began to think seriously about becoming Mr. America and unfortunately it was at this same time that I began to head down the wrong training path (though I didn't know it at the time) and to make mistakes I was to pay for later.

My first big error—and it was a whopper—was deciding to forsake my little training book and begin to train like I'd heard all the top bodybuilders trained. After all, it made sense. Those guys were my heroes. I saw their pictures in the muscle magazines. I read the articles. They said every single title winner was training six days a week, at least two hours a day. Who was I to question Steve Reeves, Armand Tanny, and Bill Pearl? As a teenager, with no real responsibilities and a great deal of energy, such a training program seemed perfectly logical and not at all demanding. I quickly became a gym rat.

And I'm not afraid to admit that I liked it. In some ways bodybuilders are like pool players who only feel really comfortable under the soft glow of the green-shaded lights in the pool-room with their pals around them. The gym is like that. It's a home with a big family. The sounds, the sweat, the joking, the lavish approval and encouragement of workout buddies, make a comfortable milieu that nurtures the weight trainer, constantly reassuring him of his strength, vigor, health, and beauty. I was so caught up in the scene that I hardly noticed that my muscular gains had slowed down considerably. I certainly didn't connect it with my marathon training methods.

But I was told that was the way it was, that it was natural, supposed to happen. I believed, but somehow it didn't seem right to me. And that was the first time I consciously remember thinking that just because a guy has a twenty-inch arm doesn't necessarily mean he knows what he's talking about. Later I was to discover that in some cases there is an inverse relationship between the size of the bicep and the size of the brain.

Still, it wasn't until four years later, when I was in the Air Force, that I began to seriously question my training practices. By that time I was up to at least eighteen hours a week and nothing discernible was happening except that I felt tired all the time. Then I began to compound my mistakes. I reasoned that if three hours a day wasn't enough time in the gym then I would spend four, five, or even more hours if necessary. Luckily for me there just weren't enough hours in the day, or enough energy in my body to handle the full-time air force job and full-time workouts. And I began to think that if developing a Mr. America physique meant giving up my entire social life and a third of my waking hours, it might not be worth the effort.

While agonizing over the very real prospect of forsaking my dream, I was introduced to Casey Viator, the 1971 Mr. America. That meeting was a fortunate turn of events for me because it completely changed my outlook on training. Casey, who was only eighteen when he won the title, and I talked a lot about training and how time and energy consuming it could be. As we talked I became more and more interested in his methods, which were very unusual for serious bodybuilders at that time. He told me he was training on an abbreviated program, fewer and shorter workouts, and he didn't think he was losing anything. It was true. He still had one of the best physiques in the country. At any rate it meant there was still hope for me and my dream.

My zeal for training reached a fever pitch following my conversation with Casey and that year I placed tenth in the Mr. America competition. I was pleased by my showing.

But soon after that I seriously injured my right shoulder in a freak accident and was forced to stop training altogether. My rampant enthusiasm reversed itself and left me in a deep depression. Having all but forgotten my dreams of becoming a top bodybuilder, I trained only intermittently for the next few years.

Finally, in 1974 I reached a point where the lack of regular training and activity got to me. I felt useless and out of shape, and I was. So for no other reason than to condition and tone myself, I started training again, but only on an abbreviated three-day-a-week, one-hour-per-session program. To my surprise and delight, I saw immediate progress. My pants and my shirts began to get tight around the muscles and my body began to resemble its previous good form. In no time I was approaching competitive condition and I was only training a few hours a week. Bodybuilding was beginning to get a lot of good publicity in 1975 and it was then I decided to get back into competition. The 1975 Mr. America contest was scheduled for July in Los Angeles but I began training (three days a week, one hour per workout) and dieting in January just to make sure I'd be in my best condition. My return to the world of competition was an auspicious one. I placed third in the Mr. America in some very tough competition.

Fired up by my good showing, I realized I was on the right track with my new training approach. True, my training represented a radical departure from traditional training principles but at that point a dogmatic preservation of bodybuilding tradition didn't interest me. What did interest me was winning the 1976 Mr. America contest. To reach that goal I set out to refine my training regime even more. At the same time I undertook some serious research.

I began reading some psychology to better understand the links between mind and body. This led to some time spent with *Sun and Steel*, Yukio Mishima's personal testament on art and action, and Shunryu Suzuki's discussions on Zen meditation and practice in *Zen Mind, Beginner's Mind*. I then read several physiology texts to learn more about the composition and function of the muscles and the nature and effects of exercise. The works of Hans Selye, Wilhelm Reich, Arthur Steinhaus, and Per-Olof Astrand became my constant companions, slowly pushing the piles of muscle magazines into the corner. At this point, too, I began to realize that proper nutrition was a lot more than just stuffing myself with protein.

Now the nutrition books moved in and the muscle magazines were stored away. Ronald Deutsch and Jean Mayer vied with Selye and the exercise physiologists for my time, and my training bag had more books than clothes in it.

I began experimenting on myself. I changed my diet a little at a time so I could determine the effects of the changes on my physical development, energy level, digestive system, mental outlook, and general well-being. I kept daily records of calorie intake broken down by macronutrients—carbohydrates, protein, and fats—and I kept a personal journal to record my physical and emotional reactions at different levels of calorie intake. At times I went as low as 500 calories a day for a period of a week or so and then worked slowly back up to 4,000 a day just to test my system's reactions.

At the same time I was experimenting with my training methods. I cut way back on the amount of time devoted to each workout. I increased my weights for each set and I worked with greater intensity, taking as little time as possible between each exercise, sometimes actually racing the clock to finish in thirty minutes or less. As I thought more about what I was reading and doing, it began to make good sense. High-intensity, short-duration training was working. The operative word seemed to be intensity.

The long-distance runner who spends hours on the track is a good example of what I'm talking about. His workouts are sometimes interspersed with sprint work, but they are generally of low intensity and long duration. The distance runner develops long, stringy muscles and a tremendous amount of stamina. The sprinter on the other hand rarely runs distances of more than a mile during training and spends most of the time in sprints of 100, 200, and 400 meters—activities that take from ten seconds to about a minute. And the sprinter has very thick, highly muscled thighs.

Short duration, high intensity. The terms kept bouncing around in my head. It soon became obvious, through experimentation and observation, that high intensity and long duration didn't make it. Either you worked out long or you worked out hard. You simply couldn't do both because the body wasn't capable of producing the necessary energy.

I began to develop a routine and soon my workouts reached such a peak of intensity that I could finish a complete training session, working all the body parts to exhaustion, in twenty-five minutes or less. Of course, this effort drained me and I wasn't able to work out at all the next day. But this, too, was beneficial. The day of rest allowed my torn muscle tissues to mend and build and within a remarkably short time I was making gains in muscle development and endurance that I never expected to achieve and never had achieved with any other training method.

My friends and competitors were as shocked as I was at my rapid development. They wanted to know how I was doing it, what my secret was. But when I explained my new routine they refused to believe me. Most of them thought it was all a show or some kind of psyching process and that I was secretly working out at home as well as in the gym. It's amazing what decades of bodybuilding indoctrination can do to the weight trainer. They just couldn't believe that less was more.

If my gym buddies had known about my diet during this period, they would have been even more shocked because it, too, defied every precept of protein-packing so dear to the hearts of all bodybuilders and to the coaches of virtually all amateur and professional sports teams. "Meat for strength" has been the battle cry since the days of the gladiators and despite stacks of scientific research reports to the contrary, it is still the battle cry. But my diet consisted of much less protein than carbohydrate and I was still building muscle. I was eating well-balanced meals of sensible size and avoiding as much excess fat as possible. I admit I was skeptical initially but the results, which totally bore out the theories of several leading nutritionists (especially Ronald Deutsch), thoroughly convinced me. That was three years ago and I'm still a believer.

So here we are. A new training method and a new diet based on the research and theories of some of the best minds in the fields of physiology, nutrition, and psychology.

Now here's what I promise. If you faithfully follow the Mentzer Method you will shed pounds of ugly fat, build needed muscle, improve your cardiovascular fitness, improve your mental outlook and your tolerance for stress, and you will achieve these gains much faster than you ever dreamed.

A word of warning. The Mentzer Method isn't a fad approach to total fitness. It involves hard work and maintenance of effort. It won't work if you don't incorporate all of its elements into your lifestyle permanently. The diet you will follow is easy and effective, the weight training will develop skeletal-muscle strength and tone but won't turn you into a freak; and contrary to some medical opinion, the workout you will get in following the Mentzer Method *will* increase your heart and lung capacity without placing any undue strain on your heart. But you have to stick with it.

Chapter 4

Myths and Realities

Before I get to the specifics of the Mentzer Method I'd like to answer some questions (before you ask them) and put to rest some of the great myths and misunderstandings that have surrounded weight training and bodybuilding for fifty years.

Question: If I work out regularly and build muscles, won't I become muscle-bound?

Answer: This certainly must be one of the oldest canards about weight training. The origins of the charge are obscure though some of it can certainly be ascribed to jealousy and "the bully on the beach gets the beautiful girl" syndrome. Mostly, though, it's a myth that has been perpetuated by word of mouth. Invariably it's the first question people ask of me and it's the primary reason some people remain reluctant to try weight training.

It's laughable really. Nobody who ever looked at the well-muscled athletic figures sculpted by Praxiteles has remarked that they look muscle-bound, nor do they think athletes who participate in track and field weight events are unable to move with speed and agility.

More than thirty years ago, Dr. Peter Karpovich of Springfield College set out to prove that weight lifters were indeed muscle-bound. He conducted a study that compared the flexibility of

competitors in the 1950 National AAU weight lifting champion-
ships to that of a group of college physical education students.
("Flexibility" is defined as the degree to which a joint is free to
move throughout its normal range of motion.) Dr. Karpovich
found that the range of motion in the joints of the weight lifters
exceeded that of the young athletes, and concluded that weight
training that involves a full range of motion contributes positively
to flexibility. In fact, the snatch lift, which calls for lifting the
weight from the floor to an overhead position in one continuous
nonstop motion, requires exceptional reflexes and tremendous
flexibility.

More recently, a study at the United States Military Academy
(USMA) at West Point found that athletes working out with
weights were able to increase their flexibility in a matter of six
weeks.

Further proof can be found in the fact that most professional
and college football teams and many baseball teams now employ
full-time weight trainers and have their own weight-training
facilities, often including Nautilus equipment. And individual
athletes in many sports regularly train with weights. They are
obviously not afraid of becoming muscle-bound and inflexible.

In his final report on the West Point study Dr. James Peterson,
the director of the project, said, "The results provide formidable
support for the contention that strength training, when properly
performed, can in fact increase flexibility."

It's not necessary to further belabor the point. You will not
become muscle-bound as a result of working out with weights.

Q: What happens to my muscles when I stop working out?
Won't they turn to fat?

A: Just as a rose is a rose, fat is fat, and muscle is muscle. They
are two distinct types of tissue and one doesn't magically turn
into the other. Viewed under a microcope, fat appears as tiny
globular balls stuck together while muscle consists of long fibrous
strands. You build muscle by exercising and you build fat by
eating.

What has prompted the "muscle-to-fat" myth is that some
bodybuilders and weight trainers, like athletes in other sports,
tend to put on weight when they stop training. This is simply
because they are eating more and exercising less. While weight

is being added in fat, the muscles, not exercised as they once were, diminish in size. They don't disappear, they just get smaller because the exercise demands that caused their growth are no longer there. At the same time, the newly added fat is beginning to cover the muscle where it once was literally muscled out, and the previously solid body begins to look flabby and fat. And it is. But muscles have not turned to fat.

In reality, the athlete must cut back on calories and tailor food intake to meet reduced activity levels. Since most people consider athletes to be more muscular than average, when they see a boxer or a football player get fat after his days of active competition are over, they assume it's muscle turning to fat.

Of course, this doesn't have to happen. Larry Scott, the first Mr. Olympia, a man many consider the greatest bodybuilder of all time, retired in 1966 after winning his second Olympia title. Scott competed at a weight of 210. In retirement his weight went down to 165 and has fluctuated through the years between 165 and 190. He was able to do this because of his knowledge of nutrition and exercise and his willingness to continue to watch his calorie intake. Now in his forties, Scott is back in competition and though he hasn't competed in thirteen years, he is in remarkable shape.

The answer to this problem, then, is to continue to watch the diet and to exercise (though you can take it a little easier). This will keep the body in shape, trim and solid, if not competitively tuned.

If you follow the Mentzer Method you won't have this type of problem at all. Don't forget, I'm not advocating that everyone work out with the idea of becoming the idol of Muscle Beach, only that the use of weight training coupled with weight control can help you develop a better-looking, healthier body. I don't expect, and don't want, everyone to try to develop super-large muscles. So, as far as I'm concerned, the muscle-turning-to-fat question is really irrelevant.

Q: Women who train with weights develop large muscles just like men, right?

A: Wrong. When contemplating the idea of using weights to develop their bodies and tone their muscles, American women immediately conjure up images of the Eastern European women who regularly excel in the Olympic weight events. The reaction invariably is, "I don't want to look like that." Well, the chances of looking like "that" even with heavy weight-training are non-existent for the average woman. The main reason is that testosterone, the male hormone responsible for muscle building, is much less prevalent in women than in men. The hefty, muscular women seen in the weight events have probably had testosterone injections which have helped them develop much larger "male-type" muscles.

What women who train with weights do develop, however, is a firm body with a tapered waist, solid buttocks, tight thighs, and flabless arms, and actually become more feminine-looking. And, of course, the added strength will improve your golf game, your tennis stroke, and your running. Both the firmed-up body and the increased strength for sports activities are extremely desirable, enhance your enjoyment of sports and life in general, and are not the least bit masculine. These are among the reasons weight training is becoming increasingly popular among women. In fact, in many areas of the country more women than men are joining health facilities including Nautilus fitness centers and gyms and spas where weight training is available.

Every day I see women training at the gym, but I've never seen any of them even begin to develop the musculature of a man. They do build strength, lose body fat, get rid of sagging triceps, double chin, creeping cellulite, and more clearly define their appearance. Remember, muscle gives curves, fat is shapeless.

Q: How about hurting myself? Won't I strain something if I train with weights?

A: *The New York Times* has cited statistics that indicate a growing percentage of pedestrian accidents appear to involve runners or joggers and traffic is only one of the hazards runners face, and probably the least dangerous. There are potholes, bicyclists, hostile pedestrians, even more hostile dogs, and of course, a wide variety of physical injuries not related to any of the foregoing, but just to the stress placed on the body by the continuous pounding—more than 1,700 hard jolts per mile. The chances of sustaining knee, ankle, leg, foot, and back injuries while jogging are incredibly high. One study has shown that if you jog regularly, your chances of sustaining some type of injury in any given twelve-month period are 80 percent.

Weight training, on the other hand, is statistically one of the safest sports around. The same study that showed a high injury rate for joggers showed a less than 1 percent chance of injury from properly conducted weight training. As in any sport, if you insist on living dangerously, weight training can be as dangerous as the next game. If you don't warm up properly, if you try to impress your friends by lifting heavier weights than you're used to, you can hurt yourself. But properly controlled weight training is among the safest methods of exercise available.

There are several reasons for this. First, if you work out in a gym, you are in a controlled atmosphere, usually with instruction and advice available, and there are always helping hands nearby for handling weights if needed. Second, your own strength is limited and your body will not be able to lift weights heavier than you can handle. Third, if something starts to strain or tighten, you can stop immediately, rest, sit down, lie down, whatever.

Weight training is also safe for the beginner and the previously sedentary adult who hasn't engaged in any sports activity in years. For one thing, it is considerably easier to monitor your pulse rate during weight training than during a fast game of tennis or racquetball or even while jogging. A monitored pulse rate is an essential element in achieving cardiovascular fitness.

Of course injuries in sports are common—tennis elbow, bruises and worse from being hit with the racquet or ball in racquetball, lower-back problems from putting too much in the golf swing—but no currently popular exercise activity matches jogging for the sheer number and variety of injuries. It amazes me that every jogging magazine and all the books on running devote a great deal of space to medical problems—how to prevent and treat injuries—while weight training and bodybuilding magazines and books rarely mention, let alone focus on, the injury question. The reason is, there are so few weight–training-related injuries that there is no point in wasting time and space to discuss them. This contrast is quite interesting to me in light of the fact that so many people think working with weights is fraught with danger.

It's also interesting that even professional runners who know the mechanics of warm-up and cool-down, as well as the basics of exercise physiology, still suffer injuries to legs, muscles, feet, tendons, and backs. While hernia and strained backs are thought to be the ultimate rewards of regular weight training, there are few such injuries and even beginnners are unlikely to suffer any injury at all. I remember, when I first started training, my father was concerned that I would rupture myself. That was always the first warning young men got from their parents. "If you try to lift too much, you'll rupture yourself," he said. Well, I've never ruptured myself, and the only injuries I've ever suffered were the result of my own eagerness and the use of improper techniques.

Of course, if you hop out of bed one morning feeling strong, rush off to the gym, grab a 300-pound barbell, and try to yank it off the floor, you'll probably end up with a sore back.

One final word. Dr. George Sheehan, jogging's philosopher-poet, glorifies the mental and physical agonies of the long-distance runner and extols the courage and fortitude necessary to overcome the pain involved. He talks of pain as a mystical, positive benefit of running. Frankly, the mysticism of pain mystifies me. It's another throwback to the Victorian ethic that says you have to suffer to get something good. Certainly, my workouts put a heavy strain on my body. There is always a certain amount of discomfort involved in physical training, but it doesn't have to be painful or injurious. Training does require work, exertion, and sweat, but there is no reason to glorify and amplify the discomfort which is minimal.

Q: What about homosexuality? Aren't a lot of weight trainers homosexual?

A: This charge is so patently false it hardly needs to be answered. There certainly are bodybuilders who are homosexual but the percentage is no greater than in the entertainment industry, in other sports, or among the general population.

This type of allegation is always found where males tend to congregate. I have spent a good portion of my life in gyms, hanging around with bodybuilders, comparing my stage of development to theirs. I like my body. I like good-looking, healthy bodies in general. But I'm not gay and few bodybuilders are. Most, in fact, are married and have families.

Yet, like the muscle-bound tag, weight trainers are thought to be gay or looked on as susceptible, as if by looking in the mirror you can catch homosexuality. Even if weight trainers were largely homosexual, I'd say, so what? These days, who cares? But, in fact, it isn't true.

The real problem gets back to the fact that men are not supposed to admire themselves, dote on their appearance, check themselves out in the mirror, wear clothes designed to show off their bodies. It's perfectly all right for women to spend hours in front of the mirror, but it's supposed to be aberrant behavior for men to enjoy doing the same thing.

Since bodybuilding is such a visual sport, the mirror is the best means of assessing progress. It is the equivalent of the runner's stopwatch. I use the mirror to check my gains and losses, to pinpoint areas where I need more work, to check for fat.

Until you develop a positive attitude toward your body and become comfortable with it you will have problems. I suppose we can blame Narcissus for this. After all, he pined away over his own image and put a word in our vocabulary that has always had negative connotations. But what weight trainers and other athletes have developed for the most part is a positive kind of Narcissism that venerates the body in a healthy way. I have a feeling that most people who don't spend some time looking at themselves in the mirror simply don't like what they see.

It's not easy to squelch old wives' tales, or put half-truths to rest. Mostly, you have to prove things to yourself, to experience them before they have any reality. I know that as soon as you begin training using the Mentzer Method you will be able to answer all of these questions for yourself.

Chapter 5

Health and Strength

In the last five years, physical fitness has become a major nondenominational religion in the United States. Louis Harris and Gallup polls show that nearly 60 percent of the nation's adults (more than 90 million people) exercise on a regular basis. This figure is more than double the number of participants indicated in a similar poll in 1961. A study financed by Great Waters of France, the Perrier people, shows that almost half of today's fitness buffs are women and that women are taking up new sports at a faster rate than men. Another survey found that a remarkable 38 percent of those fifty years old and older exercise regularly. Whatever the reasons, Americans, at long last, are discovering their bodies.

The polls, studies, and surveys aren't really necessary, though. We can easily see for ourselves that people are out and doing. Just go to the nearest park any weekend and watch the joggers vie for road room with bicyclists, roller skaters, and skate boarders. See a soccer or volleyball game, then move on to the touch football and baseball fields. On your way, check the basketball and tennis courts and the swimming pool, and be sure to watch out for flying Frisbees along the way. Sometimes it seems all 90 million people are in the park at the same time.

There is, of course, further evidence of the fitness craze all around us. Whole industries have been developed to provide for all the real and imagined needs and wants of a newly health-conscious society. Vitamin and health food stores, spas, and gyms are proliferating. Equipment manufacturers are working overtime to develop and market dozens of new, mostly useless, exercise aids. The clothing industry is churning out everything from $75 tennis shirts to running bras, and the shelves of the bookstores are crowded with health and fitness guides that promise and promise.

And like all other movements, fitness has it gurus, from Dr. George Sheehan, running's philosopher-king who tells us pain is pleasure, to bodybuilding's Arnold Schwarzenegger who equates pumping iron with the male orgasm. Sheehan and Schwarzenegger are legitimate masters of their arts, but the movement also has its share of charlatans and camp followers who have revised all the old medicine-show scams. There are the exercise practitioners who promise "A More Beautiful You (Inside and Out) in Only Ten Seconds a Week," the diet doctors who guarantee incredible weight losses even while eating your fill, the megavitamin pushers, and assorted other super salesmen, crackpots, and outright frauds all shilling their own brand of snake oil.

Remarkable results are being claimed for everything from dance exercises to vitamin regimens. If necessity is the mother of invention, fitness seems to be the father of hyperbole. When you examine some of these claims, however, the picture seems a little distorted.

For example, there is an exercise aid on the market, made of ropes and pulleys, that, along with a diet, helps you "shape" your body. When you put your legs through two loops and hold two other loops with your hands and attach the whole apparatus to a doorknob, you are able to pull the right arm and left leg up while the left arm and right leg go down. It actually helps you simulate walking. Supposedly, you can quickly lose pounds if you use the equipment for ten minutes a day. To lose weight, of course, you have to expend more calories than you take in and this system is designed to help you use calories. Well, if my pocket calculator is correct, you would have to make nearly 3,500 movements in ten minutes (that's 350 a minute or nearly 6 a second) to expend the same amount of energy you would use in walking one mile at a brisk pace. It's ridiculous because you simply can't move that fast, but even if you could, it's a tough way to burn those calories.

Then there are the megavitamin therapists. To some of these people there is no limit to the amount of a given vitamin you can use. Niacin, which supposedly supplies energy for the nerves and the brain, is particularly abused. Dosages of up to 3,000 milligrams a day are common practice, enough to provide the recommended daily allowance (RDA) for more than 200 days. Vitamin C, the pet of Dr. Linus Pauling, is even more commonly abused. He recommends up to 1,000 milligrams an hour for the common cold and at that rate, in just 24 hours, you would consume your RDA for at least one year.

But no matter. All craziness aside, the message of fitness is getting across. More people than ever are aware of their shape or lack of it. Even the cocktail party has changed. Sure, people still mill around but now they have a glass of mineral water instead of a martini and they munch raw vegetables instead of peanuts and potato chips. The chatter is different, too. It no longer centers around investments, commuting, and babysitters, but on the newest alloy in tennis racquets, the best exercise for the waistline, and the favorite in the next marathon.

Clearly the sedentary spectator has become an active and enthusiastic participant. What happened to the "average" American, long accused of being fat and lazy, mesmerized by the television set, getting exercise only during commercials and then by moving from the easy chair to the refrigerator to get another cold beer?

In many cases he or she has been born again. There are no doubt a number of interrelated reasons for the fitness trend but probably the most important is that experts in the fields of health, nutrition, psychology, and physiology are saying that exercise is good, and though they are making no promises, it looks as if regular exercise will help us live longer, happier, more energetic lives. Even the prestigious, though notably conservative, American Heart Association now says, "An exercise training program . . . can probably decrease your chances of sustaining a heart attack or having another if you have already been stricken." And they go on to say, in a pamphlet called

Exercise Your Way to Fitness and Heart Health, that "if you have a heart attack at all, it will probably be milder if you are physically fit." Finally, the AHA has taken the position that, until all the research is done, "it is at least prudent to exercise."

The prudence of exercise is fueled by the fact that cardiovascular disease is the nation's leading cause of death and disability. It is a rare person who hasn't been shocked by the news that a friend died of a heart attack at a young age. Our outrageous eating habits, our automobile lifestyle, and our inability to adapt to the stresses of life in the twentieth century, have all contributed to many serious and often lethal health problems. Almost as frequently as we hear of heart disease we hear that someone we know had a nervous breakdown or developed ulcers, has digestive problems, is hypertense, has high blood pressure, is showing allergic reactions.

But none of these problems is as frightening to the general public as the fear of sudden death from a heart attack. Indeed, the Perrier study mentioned earlier found that 75 percent of the exercising public felt that the most important type of exercise for physical fitness is that which strengthens the heart and improves blood circulation. Psychologically, 80 percent of the respondents said they feel better in general because of exercise, 53 percent indicated they are less tense, and 29 percent felt they are now better able to cope with life's pressures.

This represents a radical and rather remarkable transformation in public thinking in the last few years and signals what we can only hope is a permanent reversal of the negative attitudes toward the body and its well-being that characterized the 1960s and early 1970s. During that turbulent time, it seemed an act of pride and faith to degrade and scar the body (and the mind) by ingesting every chemical substance that came to hand while trying to support the body's basic needs on a diet of brown rice, nuts, and berries. Atrophy of the body became a national sickness during those years. If that sounds conservative, so be it. I make no apologies because I know from long experience and experimentation that the body needs and thrives on tender loving care and proper nourishment.

Fortunately, we seem to have moved away from the conscious denial of our physical selves into a new era of personal care, self-awareness, and concern for the delicate machinery of the body. I think this is a permanent trend, a healthy, positive approach to physical and mental health that will be much more than a fad.

But for physical fitness to be more than a passing fancy it must be personalized and it must become a lifestyle, part of a lifelong commitment to proper exercise and diet. We all need to develop the motivation to improve our health and our physical appearance, but to do so intelligently we also need a clear knowledge and understanding of what is required if we are to become fit and stay that way.

Based on my own experience I want to emphasize the need for accurate information. The various muscle magazines, those I grew up with in my formative years, shaped my views and attitudes about bodybuilding and nutrition, and to a large extent, they have, and still do, shape the views of the general public toward weight training and bodybuilders. What most people—in particular, weight lifters hungry for information—fail to realize is that these magazines are commercial publications, in existence primarily to sell equipment, vitamins, and gimmicks. They are not dispensers of scientific bodybuilding information in the same way that many health, diet, and fitness books are not grounded in scientific research. None of the muscle magazines I know has scientists on their editorial staffs and only rarely does M.D. appear after the name of any of their contributors. These publications do inspire young bodybuilders and they occasionally give some valid training advice, but the good is often lost in the reams of conflicting advice and opinion and sometimes dangerous nonsense.

I was as susceptible to this commercially biased hype as the next aspiring bodybuilder and consequently I wasted a lot of time, energy, and money looking for shortcuts and magic elixirs. There is a substantial amount of scientific information about bodybuilding but it is published rather randomly in a variety of texts and much of it is quite technical. It never filters down to those who can make the most use of it—the bodybuilders.

The same thing is true of most of the scores of fitness and health-related books on the market today. Many were written by people with limited knowledge or experience and no credentials. Many others are quickies, rushed to press to take advantage of some aspect of the rapidly growing fitness market. Some are literally not worth the paper they're printed on because the information they contain is erroneous, half-true, or simply a rehash that is so mundane it acts as a sleeping pill.

I'm afraid that one of the real problems with the fitness movement, and one that won't surface for some time, is that most of the exercise and diet programs now being espoused are not based on workable, sound, scientific physiological or nutritional principles and therefore will be impossible to maintain and may actually be harmful in the long run.

Sure, it's probably true that all exercise is beneficial in some way, but jogging or lifting weights can be dangerous for people with heart problems if the intensity of the exercise is not carefully monitored, and a long-term, low-carbohydrate diet may help you lose weight but it can eventually deprive your body of needed nutrients. Even stuffing yourself with vitamin A can have toxic effects.

Whether you train with weights or run marathons you have to put together a sensible, scientific program that will help you achieve the goal you set for yourself. That ultimate goal, the goal of the Mentzer Method, is total fitness.

What Is Fitness?

Fitness is as much a state of mind as a state of health, subjective as well as objective. When someone asks, "How're you feeling?" and you answer, "Terrific, real good," and you mean it, you are probably fit. If your body is in good working order and looks good, you *do* feel good, even terrific. If something is wrong, if you're a little (or a lot) overweight, irritable, easily fatigued, you know that too; and if you admit it to yourself, you're not fit, maybe "a little out of shape."

Of course, you can go to the doctor and have a physical examination in which all the tests are designed to reveal the body's vital signs. You can come away knowing that at the time of the tests you were "healthy." But more and more, we are beginning to realize that good health is not just the absence of sickness, that good health doesn't necessarily equal fitness. You can be free of disease and be badly out of shape, so badly out of shape that a sudden demand on your physical reserves can have fatal results. In fact, clinical experience has shown that more than half of the people who have suffered heart attacks have had normal resting electrocardiograms on recent examinations. Even "stress" ECG's can give false results.

No, good health doesn't necessarily equal fitness, but the opposite is usually true. If you are fit, you are in good health. You have endurance and stamina, you have plenty of energy, you sleep well, your digestion is good, and your body is operating at a state of efficiency that allows you to exercise vigorously without fatigue, and to respond to sudden physical and emotional demands with an economy of heart action and an insignificant rise in blood pressure.

What Is the Key to Fitness?

The heart is the key. Physical fitness is often defined as cardiovascular fitness, the ability of the heart's pumping action to circulate blood through the body. You are not fit if your heart is not fit and your level of fitness is determined by your heart's ability to perform its job of transporting blood and oxygen throughout the body economically and efficiently.

Fortunately, like the skeletal muscles, the heart muscle can be trained and developed through exercise. But not just any exercise. Stretching, light calisthenics, most team games, even racquetball, tennis, or handball will not produce the kind of stressful effort and create the training effect that increases cardiovascular efficiency.

Only stressful exercise—running, cycling, rowing, swimming, weight training—can enhance the ability of the heart to do its work.

Training Effect

As far back as 1931, what is now called "training effect," the amount of vigorous exercise necessary to condition the cardiovascular system, was demonstrated by a group of Scandinavian physiologists. Their experiments showed that regular exercise with an unchanging work load gradually lowered the heart rate and that by increasing the work load it became easier for the subjects to handle the amount of the original work load with a still lower heart rate. These experiments indicated that a "training effect" takes place, and that after adapting to a given load, the only way to improve further is to increase the intensity of the load.

Later experiments showed that the exact amount of intensity varies with the individual and with age but that the activity must raise the heart rate to between 60 and 80 percent of maximal aerobic power. Maximal aerobic power (or maximal oxygen intake) is that point where the heart cannot deliver oxygen to the bloodstream fast enough to create energy for exercise and that further work at that rate will result in exhaustion. To figure your maximal attainable heart rate use a base figure of 200 and subtract your age in years. So, for example, if you're thirty years old, your maximal rate will be 170 beats per minute and you will get a training effect at 60–80 percent of that rate, or by raising your pulse level to between 112 and 136 beats per minute.

This rate must then be maintained for twelve to fifteen minutes and it should be achieved three or four times per week.* It's very important to remember that physical activity is not synonymous with physical training since physical activity has to be maintained at a high level of intensity to result in the training effect. The weekend jogger, the golfer, the bowler, while exercising in the broadest sense, is not exposing the body to a training load of sufficient intensity, duration, or frequency to produce a noticeable or measurable training effect. To achieve a training

---

* Dr. Per-Olof Astrand of the Department of Physiology, Swedish College of Physical Education, maintains that maximal oxygen intake can be attained at a submaximal level of exercise and that this lower level may be sufficient as a training stimulus. Astrand says, "Practical experience has shown that work with large muscle groups for three to five minutes followed by rest or light physical activity for an equal length of time, then a further work period, etc., . . . is an effective method of training. The tempo does not have to be maximal during the work periods. It is not necessary to be exhausted when the work is discontinued. Mild exercise . . . between the heavier bursts of activity may be advantageous."

effect it is necessary to overload the body with stress greater than that experienced in the daily routine.

Why Weight Training?

Physical fitness, according to Dr. Astrand, is determined by three key elements:

1) Capacity for energy output (aerobic and anaerobic processes, and oxygen transport);

2) Neuromuscular function (muscle strength, coordination, and technique);

3) Joint mobility

Translated, this means physical fitness is a combination of cardiovascular efficiency, muscular strength, and flexibility. The Mentzer Method of weight training provides all three elements, plus a fourth—proper nutrition and weight control—that faithfully followed can help anyone achieve total fitness and a high level of health and well-being.

Athletes are often considered the finest specimens of physical fitness, and among athletes, one group—participants in the Olympic Decathlon—is considered the most fit of all. The ten events that comprise the two-day decathlon competition require a rare combination of strength, endurance, speed, flexibility, and skill. Several of the events—the shot-put, pole vault, high jump, discus, long jump, and javelin—demand speed, strength, and agility. The short dashes require sheer speed and the 1,500-meter run requires exceptional endurance. It takes years to develop the skills necessary for these events and an equal amount of time to develop the strength and endurance to excel in them. An indispensable element in a decathlon performer's training routine is weight training, because proper weight training leads to total fitness.

The human body is an integrated organism, and though we don't know yet how every part works, we do know that the whole is dependent on the sum of its parts. When one part is weakened through illness or stress, the whole body suffers. When we eat, all parts of the body are nourished. So when we talk about exercise for total fitness we shouldn't consider exercises that affect only parts of the body. It's easy enough to see that total fitness means more than just running a few laps, doing some pushups or a few calisthenics. Fitness requires more—a combination of these elements.

As an example, let's look at jogging since it's currently one of the most popular forms of exercise with more than 17 million advocates. Jogging or running is great for the legs though it doesn't build much muscle and it has very positive aerobic benefits, and, if you don't increase your calorie intake, it will help you lose weight. But jogging doesn't increase your flexibility (it may even decrease it), it does very little for the upper body and it certainly doesn't build upper-body strength. In fact, if you take a close look at the best distance runners, they are a very spare lot with a slightly unhealthy look about them, which is not to say that they don't have obvious athletic abilities. Frankly, although I do run on occasion, I am anti-jogging on two counts. I think its overall health benefits have been exaggerated and the statistics show that the injury rate is abnormally high.

At any rate, jogging fails to meet two out of three of the total fitness criteria. In fact, of the top fifteen sports activities as determined by numbers of participants, only swimming meets all three criteria for fitness, and swimming does much more for upper-body strength than for the legs. More than 50 million people participate in biking, bowling, tennis, golf, and basketball. Can 50 million Americans be wrong? I think so.

Let's examine the tenets of total fitness separately to see what they mean and how they apply to weight training.

Cardiovascular Fitness

Heart Attack! The single greatest medical problem in this country today is heart disease. Fear of heart attacks is also the reason most people exercise. Seventy-five percent of the people responding to the Perrier Fitness Study, mentioned earlier, thought the most important type of exercise for physical fitness was any exercise that would strengthen the heart and improve blood circulation.

This concern for the health of the heart, for cardiovascular fitness, is well founded. Diseases of the heart and coronary arteries kill and cripple more Americans than all other diseases combined. The numbers are shocking—more than 800,000 dead each year and many millions afflicted to some degree. It sounds more like the results of an atomic war than the toll taken by a disease. Public concern is certainly justified. Our response as individuals is another matter.

To understand the importance of cardiovascular fitness it helps to take a look at the work the heart is required to do. The heart is a large muscle with one basic function—to pump blood through the circulatory system, transporting oxygen and food nutrients to the body's tissues while removing carbon dioxide and other waste products. It fills and empties sixty to eighty times a minute when the body is at rest, pumping a little more than a quart of blood each minute. During exercise, the heart rate can increase to 130–180 or more beats a minute, forcing it to pump twenty-five to thirty quarts of blood a minute. Of course, the heart never rests, not even for a single beat, so in seventy years it beats at least 3 billion times and pumps more than 180 million quarts of blood throughout the body. Very impressive statistics.

Heart attacks are most often caused by obstructions, usually fat, in the arteries supplying blood to the heart. When these fatty deposits stop the flow of blood, that part of the heart muscle supplied by the artery dies. The more severe the blockage the more serious the problem.

What do we mean by cardiovascular fitness? The American Heart Association calls it "a state of body efficiency enabling a person to exercise vigorously for a long time period without fatigue and to respond to sudden physical and emotional demands with an economy of heartbeats and only a modest rise in blood pressure." This means the heart is pumping blood and distributing oxygen efficiently and that if necessary you can run to catch the bus without straining the pump.

This may not sound like much but it is obvious from the gruesome statistics that cardiovascular fitness is eluding a lot of us.

There are ten factors that constitute greater risk of heart disease: high blood cholesterol, high blood pressure, heredity, being male, age, diabetes, smoking, overweight, a stressful lifestyle, and inactivity. Some of these factors are out of our control. If you are a male, your risk is higher and as you approach middle-age the risks increase. These factors can't be changed. Heredity is a fact and, if you have a family history of heart problems, your risk is greater. But, on the other hand, high blood pressure and diabetes can be treated. You can stop smoking, go on a diet, start to exercise, eat fewer fatty foods, and attempt to reduce the elements of stress in your daily life. It is a real irony that seven of the risk factors in heart disease are self-inflicted.

Although it hasn't yet been proved conclusively, there is a great deal of evidence indicating that regular exercise can prevent heart attacks and reduce the incidence of heart disease. The more recent studies have shown that a regular exercise routine is usually accompanied by weight loss, the reduction of cholesterol levels, and the lowering of blood pressure. Exercise also relieves anxiety and is an effective way of eliminating the day's accumulated stress.

But just getting out and running your laps won't do the job just as weight training won't do the job if you keep on smoking or continue to include a lot of fat in your diet. To be effective, any exercise program must be totally integrated into a healthy lifestyle.

The Mentzer Method, involving high-intensity exercise in the form of weight training and a sensible program of weight control, directly attacks all of the controllable causes of heart disease.

Weight Training and Cardiovascular Fitness

When people responded to the Perrier Study by saying that *any* exercise that would strengthen the heart and improve blood circulation was important, they probably weren't thinking about weight training. To most people, weight training means the development of skeletal muscles and has nothing to do with the heart or the cardiovascular system. But what most people don't know and what most professional exercise advocates don't seem to want to admit, is that intensive weight training (like any intensive exercise involving large-muscle groups) is a valid method of developing cardiovascular fitness as well as the skeletal-muscle strength.

The critics of the cardiovascular effects of weight training are legion. Dr. Kenneth Cooper, an early proponent of aerobic training, says emphatically that conventional weight training doesn't enhance heart fitness, and other writers stoutly maintain that weight training and isometrics lead to gains in strength but have little or no effect on the cardiovascular system. The American Heart Association, which says on one hand that a program of dynamic physical exercise that involves the rhythmic use of large muscles and challenges the circulatory system (an accurate description of weight training) is good, also says weight lifting does little to promote cardiovascular fitness.

These critics may be right, though I'm not at all sure, when they talk of the conventional weight training methods of power lifters who train with heavy weights which are lifted at maximal exertion for a few repetitions and who follow their exertion with lengthy rest periods. But I think the critics are ignoring or misapplying the basic principles of exercise physiology. They have put jogging in a special category as if it had been preordained as the exclusive method of elevating the heart rate. Primitive man no doubt achieved a maximal heart rate keeping a step ahead of the saber-toothed tiger, and a training effect can be achieved by jumping rope, chopping trees, or playing hopscotch, depending on the degree of sustained effort you put into it. In reality, the heart doesn't know or care what is making it work so hard.

Dr. Per-Olof Astrand says, "Cardiac output . . . is in many types of exercise similar." He includes exercise with the arms, combined arm and leg exercises, bicycling, walking, running, and swimming. And he goes on to say that all types of "rhythmic muscular contractions will squeeze out blood from the veins" and raise the effective pressure of flow.

A cardiovascular training effect can be achieved only if an exercise is performed at a level of intensity that raises the heart rate to around 150 beats a minute and maintains that level for twelve to fifteen minutes at least three times a week.

In 1974 Dr. James Peterson, working with a group of football players at the United States Military Academy at West Point, conducted an intensive, six-week experimental program that used weight training and only weight training as a means of increasing overall physical fitness, including cardiovascular fitness.

"The results were conclusive," Dr. Peterson says in a pamphlet called *Total Conditioning*. "It was demonstrated that a strength-training program, when properly conducted, can have a positive effect on the central components of physical fitness. Contrary to widespread opinion, not only will . . . strength training produce increases in muscular strength but will also significantly improve an individual's level of cardiovascular conditioning. The data suggests that some of these cardiovascular benefits apparently cannot be achieved by any other type of training."

Dr. Peterson noted improvement on each of sixty separate measures of cardiovascular fitness including a lower and, therefore, more efficient heart rate during light, moderate, and near maximal levels of exercise. The participants even lowered their time in the two-mile run by an average of 10 percent.

My own experience with Dr. Paul DeVore, a Washington, D.C., physician specializing in weight control and physical fitness programs, was similar. My role in the privately financed research project conducted by Dr. DeVore was to supervise the exercise programs of patients who came to him for a variety of reasons including hypertension and obesity. Based on the work of physiologist Arthur Steinhaus, Dr. Peterson, and Dr. Astrand, we developed a concept we called "Cardionics," which used weight training to improve cardiovascular fitness.

Each participant was given an exercise prescription based on age, fitness level, and heart condition. Exercises were performed three times a week for eight weeks and then participants were retested. Without exception, there was a marked increase in the cardiovascular fitness level of the people in the program. One sixty-year-old man actually doubled his fitness level in only two months.

The Mentzer Method of weight training detailed in this book can produce the same kind of training effect for you.

Muscular Strength

Human beings are designed for movement. We must be active or our muscles and bones deteriorate. The size and shape of our skeletons and muscles prevent us from running as fast as a race horse or developing the strength of a bear, but in compensation, we are incomparably diverse creatures.

We move very well and we are relatively strong, and it is our muscles that provide the apparatus for both strength and movement. When the muscles contract and relax, we move, whether it's to run, throw, lift, or just write a note to the milkman. Muscular movement is the only visible evidence of the activity of the brain.

Though there are hundreds of muscles there are only three types in humans—the skeletal or voluntary type that we can see, the smooth muscles of internal body parts such as the digestive tract, and the cardiac or heart muscle.

Skeletal muscles, the only muscles that produce movement, are actually complex bundles of thousands of fibers activated by a single motor nerve fiber. These bundles join into a tendon at each end where they attach to the skeleton. The functional part of the muscle is this group of fibers. Power, whether for bursts of activity or for repetitious movements, depends solely on the size and strength of the muscles called on to make the movement.

So strength can be defined as the ability of the skeletal muscles (on command of the brain) to apply *maximal* power *one* time. This burst of strength may be used to lift a barbell, a box of groceries, or a log for the fireplace. It is easy to see the usefulness of enhanced ability to exert maximal force, that is, gaining strength by building muscle.

A few more points and we can conclude this brief physiology lesson. There are two types of muscle contractions: the kind called isometric, in which both ends of the muscle are fixed and there is no movement in the joint, and isotonic or dynamic, where the muscle varies its length. In dynamic exercise, our concern in this book, the muscle can shorten or lengthen. When it shortens, the work is called positive and when it lengthens it's called negative. Interestingly, maximal tension is produced when the muscle lengthens (negative action) and it declines as the muscle shortens.

Adults reach maximum strength between the ages of twenty and thirty. After that there is a steady decline, so that a sixty-five-year-old person is only about 80 percent as strong as he or she was at twenty or thirty. The rate of decline is greater in the leg and trunk muscles than in the arms. Women, on the average, are only about two thirds as strong as men but, women please note, strength can, and does, increase without a proportional increase in muscle size. Women can, and do, develop muscular strength with weight training but this strength won't show itself in bigger muscles.

Fortunately or unfortunately, there is only one way to increase strength and that is to train with resistance, either isometrically against a fixed object, or dynamically with weights or machines. As far as I'm concerned, weights (or specialized Nautilus equipment that uses weights) are the best and safest way to develop strength. Training with weights has at least six distinct advantages over isometrics:

1) The muscle pump (as in *Pumping Iron*) of dynamic exercise created by alternating contraction and relaxation of the muscle forces the emptying and filling of the muscle's oxygen store and forces an immediate increase in cardiac output and oxygen intake which brings about a training effect;

2) Training the oxygen-transporting system is more efficient when a large muscle mass is involved in the work;

3) It is easier to gauge your progress when you can actually see the amount of resistance (weight) you are using and increase it as necessary;

4) Dynamic work builds endurance;

5) The use of weights (whether barbells or machines) provides the positive action of lifting and the negative action of lowering, both of which are necessary to build strength;

6) Work with weights is safer because static exercise creates a very high rise in blood pressure and even moderate, localized isometric work can cause a far higher pressure build-up than dynamic movement; this is particularly important for people with heart problems.

At this point you may be saying to yourself that physical strength isn't a necessity in a society where most people don't perform any hard physical labor, but strength *is* important in our daily lives. We're not talking here about brute strength, the ability to rip a phone book in half or to move a refrigerator by yourself, but about useful strength that can benefit the housewife and the sedentary, or even the active, executive. Today, a growing number of corporations are recommending weight training for their executive personnel and more than 400 firms have gone so far as to install their own supervised exercise facilities.

The reasoning is simple—corporate managers recognize that the health of their business depends on the physical health of key employees. Experience has proved that such programs more than pay for themselves in greater productivity, and reduced absenteeism and disability. The executive who develops his or her physique and increases strength works with added confidence and is better able to handle the stress and frustration of corporate and everyday life.

For the housewife, whose day is taken up with chores that often require lifting and strenuous movement, the development of greater physical strength and endurance will make all tasks easier, less stressful and energy draining. And weight training does something no other form of exercise can do—it makes you look better. There's not one of us who wouldn't like to look better.

For the average person, weight training is a highly useful exercise for building strength for activities that are not related to lifting weights, but for the competitive athlete, strength is of great importance to top performance.

Until quite recently, strength has been a vastly underrated aspect of athletic performance. But in the past several years, thanks largely to the work of Dr. Peterson at West Point and others, physical educators, coaches, and athletes themselves have become increasingly aware of the importance of strength whether they are shot putters, sprinters, swimmers, football players, or skiers. There seems finally to be a realization among those responsible for developing and training athletes that, given two competitors of roughly equal talent and skill, the stronger athlete will almost always win. Dr. Peterson concludes, "For the coach and the athlete, the implication [of the importance of weight training] is clear: These subjects could perform at a more efficient rate for a longer period of time. In the athletic arena, where contests are frequently decided by inches or other fractions, such training could play an important role."

Now, most professional sports teams and college athletic departments, and even many high schools, employ full-time strength coaches and have installed weight rooms in a concerted effort to build the strength and endurance of their charges. Weight training is "in" for competitive athletes and it is equally valid for the weekend or part-time athlete. With weight training you will be able to run farther and faster, hit the ball harder, ski with better form and endurance, and in general, add a sense of vitality and a feeling of vigor to everything you do.

Flexibility

As I said in Chapter 2, bodybuilding and weight training have suffered under the charge that if you train hard with weights you will build muscle and develop strength at the expense of flexibility and mobility and eventually become muscle-bound. The dictionary still defines muscle-bound as "having stiff, over-developed muscles, usually as the result of excessive exercise." Since running forty miles a week could be called excessive exercise, the definition is wrong on that count, and second, over-developed muscles are not stiff; *unused* muscles are stiff.

Despite the dictionary, I think the muscle-bound myth can finally be put to rest. The strange thing is that it didn't happen long ago. The examples have certainly been there for all to see. I remember seeing photographs of John Grimek, one of the most highly developed men of all time, doing a back flip into a split position after being named Mr. Universe at the age of forty. Among the super bodybuilders, Franco Columbu was a lightweight boxer; Mike Katz, a former Mr. America, played football for the New York Jets; and Lou Ferrigno (the Incredible Hulk) was an all-around athlete in high school and placed fourth in the "Superstars" competition competing against athletes from all sports. And no one has ever accused track and field's weight-event athletes of being muscle-bound since the key to winning performance in the shot put, discus, and javelin is strength, speed, and agility.

There is also solid, scientific proof that flexibility is not limited but is actually increased by weight training. Astrand's work has shown that the limiting factor for flexibility is often the length of the muscles and that training that produces a lengthening of these muscles will increase joint flexibility. He also has shown that regular exercise causes increased strength in ligaments and tendons and reduces the danger of injury. On the other hand, if stretching does not take place, the muscle shortens causing a loss of flexibility.

Dr. Peterson's report on his West Point weight-training program says, "The fear that 'tightened' muscles result in a lack of flexibility undoubtedly accounts for much of the superstition and misconception regarding the relationships between strength training and flexibility. The truth of the matter is that, with proper training methods, normal flexibility will not only be unaffected, but may even be increased by strength training."

Peterson's test results on USMA football players showed that in six weeks his experimental group improved on flexibility measurements by an average of nearly 11 percent while the control group (not using weights) gained less than 1 percent.

More recently, Peterson conducted a second study, in conjunction with the admission of women cadets to West Point. Weight training was part of the fitness program for the women and the results showed that in the seven-week training period upper-body strength and general endurance increased and the development of levels of flexibility were higher than the national average.

I'm not surprised at the results of either of these studies. When muscles are worked through their full range of motion they remain flexible around the joints. There is no relationship between muscular size and flexibility. It is the method used to develop the muscles that determines flexibility; therefore, exercises that involve stretching will increase flexibility. Prolonged exercises that do not provide stretching—running, for example—will not increase flexibility. It is this inflexibility that results in pulls and tears, knots and soreness.

The Mentzer Method is designed to stretch all the muscles and will actually increase your flexibility at a rate that will surprise you.

Chapter 6

There's No Secret to
Weight Control

At this point I've talked only about weight training and its benefits for your cardiovascular system, your skeletal-muscle strength, and your flexibility. Weight training, though, is only part of the Mentzer Method of achieving *total* fitness.

As I see it, the other side of the fitness coin—nutrition and weight control—is equally important to total fitness. It's a contradiction in terms to think that you're fit if you're overweight. And if you're overweight by even a couple of pounds, exercise alone won't help reduce those bulges. Exercise is an important factor in weight control because only muscular work can cause an increase in energy expenditure. But there are no magic exercises.

This means diet is also an important factor. Not just a few days at a time, not fasting one day a week, but a commitment to a permanent state of weight control.

But don't get nervous. I'm not talking about total starvation, eating only predigested protein, forcing down grapefruit and chopped anchovies for all three meals, nor am I talking about the Scarsdale, Atkins, or any of the other "fad" diets. I'm talking about permanent, not temporary, weight control. And I think permanent weight control is considerably easier than dieting.

I use the word "fad" in referring to diets because they seem to sweep across our consciousness like comets, leaving a trail of disappointed and frustrated dieters and a gaggle of authors with overweight bank accounts. There are literally scores of diets on the market and most of them will help the diligent person lose some weight, even as much as the fabled "14 pounds in 14 days" promised by one of them.

The problem is the long pull, keeping the weight off. The average person, satisfied with the instant gratification of dropping a few quick pounds (mostly water), is easily appeased and goes right back to the eating habits that helped create the overweight problem in the first place. How many times have you heard this one? "That XYZ Diet is great. I lost six pounds the first week." You never hear about the second week because the six pounds came right back. Why? You can't change your eating habits unless your food intake is balanced. This means the right percentage of carbohydrates, fats, and protein, a combination that supplies the body with all the nutrients it needs to function properly without severe deprivation. Most of the popular diets are unbalanced, unsatisfying, sometimes unhealthy, and usually downright boring. You can't stick with them.

The Mentzer Method is different. It's easy to follow. It doesn't require a weekly trip to the pharmacy or health-food store to pick up expensive pills or unneeded vitamin and mineral supplements. It doesn't deprive you of carbohydrates, fats, or proteins. The Mentzer Method is a straightforward combination of a well-balanced diet with reduced calorie intake.

I call it the Mentzer 3,500 Weight-Control Program and it's based on the body's own formula for weight control:

Energy Intake Minus Energy Output Equals Weight Gain (or Weight Loss).

It actually couldn't be more simple. If you take in more energy in the form of food than you use in the normal day's activities, then you will gain weight. If, on the other hand, you take in less than you use, you will lose weight. This translates to eating less (though it doesn't have to be a lot less) and exercising more (as few as fifteen walking steps use one calorie). To make use of the Mentzer 3,500 Weight-Control Program, it's first necessary to know the body's real caloric needs.

The BMR—How Much Does the Body Need?

The body is like a machine, more complicated and sensitive than any man-made implement, but a machine nevertheless, and like most machines it needs fuel to operate. This fuel comes from food. What we put in our mouths is synthesized in a variety of complex chemical processes and is then used as fuel for basic biological work. This basic work—all the involuntary activity that keeps the machinery going—is called the basal metabolism. The speed at which this process operates for each individual is called the basal metabolic rate (BMR). The BMR is the basic level of the body's daily energy needs and these needs are substantial.

But the BMR is only part of the story. Our body motors don't just run on idle all the time, so our other activities, from knitting to sprinting—the voluntary things we do each day—require still more energy. This energy all comes from calories.* Your total calorie needs are based on your own personal BMR plus your daily energy needs for voluntary activity.

It is essential to know this total if you are to control your weight. Here's a simple, accurate way to find your BMR and your total daily maintenance level.

If you're a man, add a zero to your present weight and then add twice your weight. So, for example, if you weigh 150, your BMR would be 1,800 (150 with an extra 0 equals 1,500, plus twice 150, or 300, equals 1,800). If you're a 125-pound woman, add a zero to your weight and then add your weight (125 with an added 0 equals 1,250 plus 125 equals 1,375). Next, this figure must be adjusted for age since people tend to be less active after age twenty.

Adjust the BMR for age by subtracting 2 percent for each decade of age. If you're thirty, subtract 6 percent; if you're forty, 8 percent, and so on. Using these examples, the 150-pound, thirty-year-old man would have an adjusted BMR of 1,692 (1,800 minus 6 percent [108] equals 1,692). The woman's BMR at thirty would be 1,293 (1,375 minus 6 percent [82] equals 1,293). The body's energy balance is remarkably delicate so it's important to be very careful about energy intake as you age. If, as you grow older, you cut back your energy use even 150 calories a day and con-

* For convenience, everyone uses the word "calorie" but food doesn't actually contain calories, it contains energy potential and that *potential* is measured in calories. The common terminology is that food supplies calories that are turned into energy or fuel for the body.

2087
63 0ar 30%
―――――
2717

3237.5
-2717
―――――
520 ÷ 2 = 260
∴ 2717 + 260 = 2977 ≟ 3000

tinue to eat in the same way, you'll gain more than a pound a month.

Now make an upward adjustment that will reflect your activity level, the cost in calories of your daily voluntary movement. Remember this activity can range from very heavy physical exertion (athletes in training, manual labor, climbing) to very light work (sitting, sewing, driving). But on the average, unless you're extremely active or passive, this rate of consumption can be figured at 30 percent of the age-adjusted BMR.* So once again, taking the 150-pound man as an example, his total daily need will be 2,200 (BMR 1,692 + 30 percent or 508 = 2,200). The 125-pound woman's rate will be 1,681 (BMR 1,293 + 30 percent or 388 = 1,681). Since calorie counting and BMR figures are not absolutely exact, it's easier to round off the final figure to the nearest zero.**

The Mentzer 3,500 Weight-Control Program

First let me say that I make no claim to having discovered the 3,500 Weight-Control Program. The concept has been well known for a long time and it is a matter of such basic arithmetic it's a wonder to me we don't all live by the numbers. What I'm going to tell you is how to use the 3,500 Weight-Control Program (in conjunction with the Mentzer Method weight training exercises) to lose weight and keep it off permanently.

This number—3,500—is the absolute key to weight control. It represents the number of calories in a pound of fat. You can forget everything else you've ever read about dieting. From this point on, 3,500 is the bottom line.

Going back to the simple arithmetic of weight loss (Energy Intake Minus Energy Expenditure Equals Weight Gain or Loss), it's easy to see that you have to consume 3,500 extra calories, over and above your daily needs (BMR plus energy expenditure), to gain a pound of body fat and you have to cut your consumption

* For those who want a more exact figure, there is an energy expenditure chart on the following page.
** Some nutritionists suggest using an overall figure of 17.5 calories per pound of body weight per day for men and 15.5 for women. This will give you a slightly higher total and you may want to begin your weight control program using this formula.

Calorie-Expenditure Chart

ACTIVITY	CALORIES PER MINUTE [*]
Driving a car	.50
Typing, sewing, standing	.60
Heavy housework	.90
Walking easily	1.60
Bicycling easily	2.10
Dancing moderately	2.70
Skating moderately	3.20
Swimming moderately	3.20
Walking fast	3.20
Walking uphill or upstairs	4.80
Tennis	5.10
Jogging	7.00
Bicycling fast	7.60
Weight training intensely	8.00
Swimming fast	8.00
Running fast	8.90

[*] The figures given are for men weighing 150 pounds and women weighing 125 pounds. This listing is a compilation of various research findings and should be considered approximations.

by 3,500 calories to lose a pound of stored fat. How much is 3,500 calories? It's seventeen waffles without syrup and butter, ten cups of spaghetti and meatballs, ten cups of chili with beans, thirty-five donuts, or a whole pecan pie. It's a lot. In fact, 3,500 calories is more than most of us eat in an entire day. If you regularly consume 2,500 calories a day and maintain your weight, you'd have to eat five donuts a day or two and a half waffles a day for a week to compile the extra 3,500 calories needed to add a pound of fat. With this in mind, it's easier to see why large, permanent weight losses (or gains, for that matter) are impossible in a short period of time. Let's say your daily needs total 2,500 calories. Obviously, at that rate of consumption, if you ate nothing at all you couldn't lose a pound of fat a day, and you'd have to eat a hefty 6,000 calories to gain a pound a day.

To lose weight you need to cut back your total daily calorie intake but you don't have to cut that much. Sensibly, if you continue to eat a variety of foods (essentially your current diet) and cut back from 2,500 calories to 2,000 per day—a reduction of only 500—you could lose a pound a week (500 per day × 7 days = 3,500). Not bad, and not that difficult either. At that modest rate, in seventy days, a little more than two months, you could lose ten pounds and keep it off because the loss was accomplished slowly and painlessly without really depriving yourself of anything.

Now, if you combine this reduction in calories with the additional energy expenditure required by the Mentzer Method exercises, you can increase the speed of weight loss because you'll be increasing your calorie deficit. A reduction of 500 calories per day plus an energy expenditure of approximately 300 calories three times a week will total a 4,400-calorie deficit each week and result in the loss of two and a half pounds in two weeks.

It sounds easy and it is easy if you can discipline yourself and stay with it. At best, the ability of human beings to regulate their food intake is very poor, and sedentary people almost always eat more than they need. Exercise is important to weight control, it counts just as much as calories count. Exercise tends to decrease appetite, and the rise in body temperature that occurs during exercise also inhibits hunger. Physiologists and nutritionists agree that the intensity of the exercise is also important in caloric cost, and only muscular work, in whatever form, uses the body's energy. Sitting and thinking about exercise won't do a thing but help broaden your behind.

In the Mentzer 3,500 Program, calories and only calories count, so here's how I suggest you keep track. Before you begin the program, weigh yourself (an ordinary bathroom scale will do but use the same scale each time), buy an inexpensive calorie-counting book at the drug store, and a pocket-sized note pad. For the next five days eat your normal diet, but record everything you eat, and I mean everything. Don't forget that piece of chewing gum or the milk in your coffee. Every time you pop something in your mouth write it down along with the quantity. At the end of each day, use the calorie counter and total the calories consumed. If you've been a faithful recorder, you'll probably be surprised and shocked at the sheer number of entries. Most people eat much more and much more often than they think they do. At the end of five days, add the daily figures and divide by five. This will give you a daily average. (See chart on page 60.)

Now weigh yourself a second time. You may have gained or lost a pound but if you have continued to eat the way you normally do, you should have remained at about the same weight as when you started counting. This means the calorie figure you have in your hand is your current level of caloric intake. If you didn't gain or lose, it also represents your total daily needs at your current weight.

If you want to reduce *your* figure, you must reduce *that* figure. That's all there is to it. Reduce your calorie intake, add exercise, and watch your weight go down and stay down. The number is 3,500. Learn to live with it from now on.

For the first few weeks I'd advise you to continue to keep a daily calorie count. It's a good incentive. You'll soon know the calories of most items so you won't have to keep referring to the book and you'll begin to make those trade-offs that make it possible to hit your daily target, but with a variety of foods. I do it all the time. I'll trade a dip of ice cream for two apples any day and I know my body doesn't care what kind of food is supplying its energy as long as its needs are being met. Of course, this doesn't mean you should try to live on ice cream or donuts or brown rice. For total nutrition your diet must be well balanced.

The Well-Balanced Diet

It may be simplistic to say that the well-balanced diet is "a little bit of everything," but in fact, that's exactly what it is. Nutritionists have divided foods into four groups based on similarities in nutritive value and their role in the diet. A well-balanced diet includes several servings from each group every day. Here's how they break down:

> • Meat Group—Two or more servings of meat, fish, poultry, or eggs. Nuts and beans can be substituted.*

* Serving size is average (i.e., three ounces of meat), and does not include gravies or sauces. The grains should not be included in cakes, pies, or other sweets. This does not mean that you shouldn't have gravy on your potatoes or cake for dessert, just that such items generally add only calories and little of nutritive value.

Calorie Journal

STARTING DATE_____ WEIGHT_____ MAINTENANCE LEVEL_____

DATE	BKFST.	LUNCH	DINNER	SNACKS	MISC.	TOTAL	WEIGHT

- Vegetables and Fruits—Four or more servings.
- Milk Group—Two or more glasses of milk or servings of cheese, butter, or ice cream.
- Breads and Cereals—Four or more servings.

The basic four are not the be all and end all of eating and nutrition but they are a reliable guide to well-balanced consumption. They are analyzed in much greater detail in books devoted to nutrition (not diet books) and individual adjustments can be made to suit your basic needs, your additional needs for energy consumption (exercise and pregnancy can increase the total amount of food you eat and consequently the nutrients you ingest), products available in your part of the country, and your lifestyle.

A person who eats a diet that includes most of the foods in the basic four each day should not need vitamin or mineral supplements of any kind.

The nutrients provided in the well-balanced diet include:

Macronutrients

There are four macronutrients: carbohydrates, fat, protein, and water. They are the body's only important source of energy and they are therefore used in great quantities. The carbohydrates, much maligned by the diet doctors, are the body's main source of fuel. They're stored in the muscles and liver in the form of energy-giving glycogen. Fats, stored in the muscles, under the skin, and around body organs, are the second-best source of energy. Protein, though it enjoys the best publicity, is a poor energy provider at any time, and the body has no way of storing it. Water may be the most important of all the nutrients. We can live for some time without protein, fat, and carbohydrate, but we only last a few days without water.

Let's take a closer look.

Carbohydrates—Carbohydrates are chemical compounds of sugar, starches, and cellulose (fiber) containing carbon, hydrogen, and oxygen. The most important carbohydrate is glucose, the body's primary energy source. The sugar molecules in food are called monosaccharides (individual molecules), disaccharides (pairs), and polysaccharides (three or more). The body can only absorb monosaccharides so it chemically breaks down di- and polysaccharides into the usable form—monosoccharides. Glucose, fructose, and galactose are the only monosaccharides that find their way to the liver, where fructose and galactose are converted to glucose and used for energy. Sugar, because it contains readily usable glucose, is absorbed into the bloodstream very quickly. Starches need to be broken down and are absorbed more slowly.

Interestingly, the original source of the glucose doesn't matter in the slightest. Glucose is glucose whether it comes from an ice cream soda or mashed potatoes. As a source of energy, however, pure sugar or honey are poor choices. They are absorbed immediately and may give a "rush" of energy, but there is no lasting effect. The more complex carbohydrates found in such starches as potatoes and peas take longer for the body to process and provide a longer lasting energy source.

Ordinarily, there is less than a quarter of an ounce of glucose available in the bloodstream at any one time. But the body has ten to twelve ounces more in storage in the heart and muscle tissue. This reserve energy is used during prolonged exercise. Roughly 50 percent of the daily calorie intake should consist of carbohydrates.

Fats—Fats, or lipids, are chemical compounds that don't dissolve in water. Most fats (about 98 percent) are called triglycerides, of which some are saturated and come from animals and some are unsaturated and come from plants. Fats are very caloric—about 3,500 calories per pound, as you'll recall. This is more than twice the calorie density of carbohydrates. Low-fat diets are very effective for trimming the pounds but much of the fat consumed daily is hidden (in meat, milk, cheese, and nuts) and difficult to eliminate without excluding other valuable nutrients as well. Fat should make up less than 35 percent of your daily diet, especially if you're concerned about the potentially damaging effects cholesterol may have on the cardiovascular system.

Protein—Protein is the organic material that, next to water, is the primary structural material of the body's cells and tissues. There are about twenty amino acids in protein and at least nine of these (the "essential" amino acids) have to come from the daily diet. But just as the body doesn't care where it gets its glucose, it isn't concerned about the source of its protein. In other words, beans are as good as meat.

Nutritionist Ronald Deutsch feels that "protein has become the dietary lure to which the consumer consistently rises, like a hungry trout on a quiet morning." There is truth in what he says. It's a fact, of course, that protein is absolutely essential for growth and repair of the body's tissues, but it has yet to be proven that more than enough of any essential element of nutrition is better than merely enough.

The average adult needs about 70 grams of protein per day for normal growth and development. This translates to about nine ounces of broiled hamburger, which also contain about 30 grams of fat. Yet I know bodybuilders who eat 500 grams of protein a day thinking it will help them gain additional muscle. The protein they're eating obviously contains calories just as fats and carbohydrates do. The extra protein doesn't help. In fact, it hurts, because the excess is stored as fat, even when the extra protein comes from steak. You'd need to eat a little more than five pounds of steak to get the 500 grams of protein. Unfortunately, this amount of meat contains more than 8,000 calories and about 675 grams of fat. Think of the exercise necessary to work off those extra calories. I'd estimate it at more than fifteen hours of intense work. With the cost of meat what it is, this type of useless excess is expensive in more ways than one. If your daily diet consists of 15 percent protein you have nothing to worry about.

Water—The importance of water is obvious when you consider that the body is 60 percent water. Water not only contains valuable minerals but also it acts as a lubricator, a shock absorber between cells, a digestion aid, and is the body's principal means of cooling, performing the essential job of maintaining the body's normal temperature.

In the course of an average day the body loses water steadily, though much of this loss (about 50 percent) is unseen. On a hot day it's not uncommon to lose five to eight quarts of fluid which, of course, must be replaced either by drinking liquids (again, it doesn't matter what you drink—with the exception of alcohol—nor does the temperature of the drink matter) or through the food normally consumed. A surprising amount of seemingly solid food contains a high percentage of water. Meats can be as much as half water while most fruits and vegetables are at least 70 percent water.

If you get thirsty while exercising, don't hesitate to drink fluids. Your body is trying to tell you something. The idea that the athlete shouldn't drink while practicing has been discarded. Drinking fluids during exercise does not cause cramps—an old but persistent error. Remember though, immediate weight-loss during exercise is almost all fluid. Exercise eventually cuts into the fat content of your body but it takes time for this effect to appear.

Micronutrients

Vitamins—Vitamins are organic substances that play a major role in the control of the body's metabolic processes. They help to process the macronutrients—carbohydrates, fats, and protein—and serve as aids to the body's own self-produced enzymes (forming coenzymes), which function as biochemical catalysts.

The body cannot manufacture its own vitamins so they must be obtained from the diet. This is not at all difficult if you're eating a well-balanced diet because the daily vitamin requirement is ⅛ teaspoon. Interestingly, though nutritionists agree that vitamins are essential to good health, there is little agreement on which vitamins (if any) are most important, the proper dosage, or who needs them. (See chart on pages 66 and 67.)

It does seem clear, however, that vitamins in any amount do not cure disease or provide extra health protection. Ronald Deutsch says, "In extra doses, used essentially as medicines, vitamins and minerals cure scarcely anything except deficiencies in vitamins and minerals." This, of course, includes the extravagant claims made for vitamin C (as a cold cure) and vitamin E (as a hedge against aging).

Deutsch's views are underlined in a report by the American Psychiatric Association which concludes, "The results and claims

RECOMMENDED DAILY DIETARY ALLOWANCES (RDA'S) *

(Designed for the maintenance of good nutrition of practically all healthy persons in the United States.)

Sex-age category	Persons Age Years From	To	Weight Kilograms	Pounds	Height Centimeters	Inches	Food energy Calories	Protein Grams	Minerals Calcium Milligrams	Phosphorus Milligrams	Iron Milligrams	Vitamin A International units	Thiamin Milligrams	Riboflavin Milligrams	Niacin Milligrams	Ascorbic acid Milligrams
Infants	0	0.5	6	14	60	24	kg x 117 / lb x 53.2	kg x 2.2 / lb x 1.0	360	240	10	1,400	0.3	0.4	5	35
	0.5	1	9	20	71	28	kg x 108 / lb x 49.1	kg x 2.0 / lb x 0.9	540	400	15	2,000	.5	.6	8	35
Children	1	3	13	28	86	34	1,300	23	800	800	15	2,000	.7	.8	9	40
	4	6	20	44	110	44	1,800	30	800	800	10	2,500	.9	1.1	12	40
	7	10	30	66	135	54	2,400	36	800	800	10	3,300	1.2	1.2	16	40
Males	11	14	44	97	158	63	2,800	44	1,200	1,200	18	5,000	1.4	1.5	18	45
	15	18	61	134	172	69	3,000	54	1,200	1,200	18	5,000	1.5	1.8	20	45
	19	22	67	147	172	69	3,000	54	800	800	10	5,000	1.5	1.8	20	45
	23	50	70	154	172	69	2,700	56	800	800	10	5,000	1.4	1.6	18	45
	51+		70	154	172	69	2,400	56	800	800	10	5,000	1.2	1.5	16	45
Females	11	14	44	97	155	62	2,400	44	1,200	1,200	18	4,000	1.2	1.3	16	45
	15	18	54	119	162	65	2,100	48	1,200	1,200	18	4,000	1.1	1.4	14	45
	19	22	58	128	162	65	2,100	46	800	800	18	4,000	1.1	1.4	14	45
	23	50	58	128	162	65	2,000	46	800	800	18	4,000	1.0	1.2	13	45
	51+		58	128	162	65	1,800	46	800	800	10	4,000	1.0	1.2	12	45
Pregnant							+300	+30	1,200	1,200	2+18	5,000	+.3	+.3	+2	60
Lactating							+500	+20	1,200	1,200	18	6,000	+.3	+.5	+4	80

* From *Nutritive Value of Foods*, U. S. Department of Agriculture, Washington, D.C., Sept., 1978.

A GUIDE TO THE VITAMINS

VITAMIN	BEST SOURCES	MAIN ROLES	DEFICIENCY SYMPTOMS
A	Liver; eggs; cheese; butter, fortified margarine and milk; yellow, orange and dark green vegetables (e.g., carrots, broccoli, squash, spinach).	Formation and maintenance of skin and mucous membranes; bone growth; vision; reproduction; teeth.	Night blindness; rough skin and mucous membranes; no bone growth; cracked, decayed teeth; drying of eyes.
Thiamin (B1)	Pork (especially ham); liver; oysters; whole grain and enriched cereals, pasta and bread; wheat germ; brewers yeast; green peas.	Release of energy from carbohydrates; synthesis of nerve-regulating substance.	Beriberi: mental confusion; muscular weakness; swelling of heart; leg cramps.
Riboflavin (B2)	Liver, milk, meat, dark green vegetables, whole grain and enriched cereals, pasta and bread, mushrooms.	Release of energy to cells from carbohydrates, proteins and fats; maintenance of mucous membranes.	Skin disorders, especially around nose and lips; cracks at mouth corners, eyes very sensitive to light.
Niacin (B3)	Liver; poultry; meat; tuna, whole grain and enriched cereals, pasta and bread; nuts, dried beans and peas. Made in body from amino acid tryptophan.	Works with thiamin and riboflavin in energy-producing reactions in cells.	Pellegra: skin disorders, especially parts exposed to sun; smooth tongue; diarrhea; mental confusion; irritability.
Pyridoxine (B6)	Whole grain (but not enriched) cereals and bread; liver; avocados; spinach; green beans; bananas.	Absorption and metabolism of proteins; use of fats; formation of red blood cells.	Skin disorders; cracks at mouth corners; smooth tongue; convulsions; dizziness; nausea; anemia; kidney stones.
Cobalamin (B12)	Liver; kidneys; meat; fish; eggs; milk; oysters.	Building of genetic material, formation of red blood cells, functioning of nervous system.	Pernicious anemia: anemia; degeneration of peripheral nerves.

Vitamin	Sources	Function	Deficiency Symptoms
Folic acid (Folacin)	Liver; kidneys; dark green leafy vegetables; wheat germ; brewers yeast.	Assists in forming body proteins and genetic material; formation of hemoglobin.	Anemia with large red blood cells; smooth tongue; diarrhea.
Pantothenic acid	Liver; kidneys; whole grain bread and cereal; nuts; eggs; dark green vegetables; yeast.	Metabolism of carbohydrates, proteins and fats; formation of hormones and nerve-regulating substances.	Not known except experimentally in man: vomiting; abdominal pain; fatigue; sleep problems.
Biotin	Egg yolk; liver; kidneys; dark green vegetables; green beans. Made in intestinal tract.	Formation of fatty acids; release of energy from carbohydrates.	Not known except experimentally in man: fatigue; depression; nausea; pains; loss of appetite.
C (Ascorbic acid)	Many fruits and vegetables, including citrus, tomato, strawberries, melon, green pepper, potato, dark green vegetables.	Maintenance of health of bones, teeth, blood vessels; formation of collagen, which supports body structure; antioxidant.	Scurvy; gums bleed; muscles degenerate; wounds don't heal; skin rough, brown and dry; teeth loosen.
D	Milk; egg yolk; liver, tuna, salmon. Made on skin in sunlight.	Essential for normal bone growth and maintenance of strong bones.	Rickets (in children): retarded growth; bowed legs; malformed teeth; protruding abdomen. Osteomalacia (in adults): bones soften, deform and fracture easily; muscular twitching and spasms.
E	Vegetable oils; margarine; whole grain cereal and bread; wheat germ; liver; dried beans; green leafy vegetables.	Formation of red blood cells, muscle and other tissues; prevents oxidation of vitamin A and fats.	Breakdown of red blood cells. Symptoms in animals (reproductive failure, liver degeneration, muscular dystrophy, etc.) not seen in man.
K	Green leafy vegetables; vegetables in cabbage family; milk. Made in intestinal tract.	Essential for normal blood clotting.	Hemorrhage (especially in newborns).

of the advocates of megavitamin therapy have not been confirmed." The APA panel found "the massive publicity which they [megavitamin therapists] promulgate via radio, the lay press and popular books . . . to be deplorable."

It is possible that vegetarians, food faddists, people on low-calorie diets, and very fussy eaters may not get the United States Recommended Daily Allowance of vitamins (see chart on page 65). But even this is unlikely (and easily rectified with a multivitamin supplement) because the fat soluble vitamins—A, D, E, and K—are stored in the body's fat and don't need to be consumed daily. The water soluble vitamins—C and eight B vitamins—should be consumed daily but they are very easy to acquire even in a moderately well-balanced diet.

One other point. Vitamins do not provide energy and there is absolutely no need to increase your vitamin intake even during heavy exercise.

Minerals—Minerals are chemicals found in the soil and passed to humans through plants and animals. They are vital to life processes but only in small quantities. They activate hormones, prevent anemia, and are essential in controlling heartbeat and muscle contraction. The most important, or at least those minerals needed in the largest amounts, are sodium, magnesium, calcium, and potassium. Other minerals, including iron, cobalt, and iodine, are needed in trace amounts. (See chart on page 65.) Most minerals can be obtained from the daily diet if that diet includes vegetables, fruits, grains, and dairy products.

Diets and Why They Work

In the years I've been training I've tried at least fifty kinds of diets and lost a cumulative total of hundreds of pounds. I've gobbled vitamin pills, gone down starvation road, stuffed protein one week and carbohydrates the next, and I've eaten obnoxious mixtures I don't even want to think about.

I still vividly remember one diet I tried when I was training for my first Mr. America contest. It's a constant reminder to me that diet gimmicks are diet gimmicks.

A friend told me about an avocado diet that, he said, helped

him lose ten pounds in one week. The diet consisted solely of
avocados sprinkled with a little oil and vinegar for taste. Being
a true believer in those days, I went to the market, stocked up
on a week's worth of avocados, and started eating them four or
five times a day. Yes, I lost weight. But it was mainly because
after three days I felt as green as the Incredible Hulk, inside
and out. I couldn't eat another avocado, or anything else, for
that matter, for three more days. In one sense the diet worked.

Of course, I gained back all the lost weight, only about six
pounds, in less time than it took to lose it.

Most diets work in the short run because, whatever they may
promise about eating all you want, their main trick is to get
you to eat less. The big "secret" is a reduction in your calorie
consumption, often by excluding one of the macronutrients,
usually carbohydrates (bread, potatoes, pasta, desserts). Psychologically, most such diets quickly become boring and you tend to
eat even less than the diet's suggested allowance. What the
Stillman, Atkins, and most other diets do is reduce the carbohydrate intake to below 60 grams a day. This causes weight loss.

Here's why. Carbohydrates are the body's main source of
energy. The low-carbohydrate diet forces the body to reach into
itself for substitute forms of fuel—some of its protein and stored
fat. This shift in internal chemical processes results in more waste
products. These wastes activate the kidneys and they, in turn,
respond by getting rid of the waste. This reduces the body's
water content. This loss can conceivably add up to ten pounds
in a week, but it's almost all fluid. Since fat contains very little
water, you aren't losing fat.

Ronald Deutsch puts the problem in perspective in his book
Realities of Nutrition. Deutsch says, "To give some idea of how
much stored energy fat represents, consider the 'typical' young
American woman, at five feet five inches and 128 pounds. A
little over 25 of those pounds are in fat. And this much fat has
enough energy potential to meet all the woman's needs for
about 45 days, if she gets no food at all."

Your body has a tremendous amount of energy in reserve even
if you aren't overweight. It obviously takes a severe and prolonged energy shortage to make any progress against excess fat.

What Is Overweight?

As I've said, you can't be overweight by even a few pounds and be totally fit because that few pounds is excess fat. The body has a sophisticated system of storing fuel for later use—keeping the tank filled. That extra fuel, over and above the combined BMR/Energy Expenditure rate, is converted to fat (the few pounds mentioned above). The body is designed to store a certain amount of fat for energy reserve (it's an extremely compact fuel supply providing twice as much energy per calorie as either protein or carbohydrate), for insulation, for padding, and for the lean times. But these days, in this country at least, there are relatively few lean times so most of us store fat, fat, and more fat. This excess serves no useful purpose, it's potentially harmful, and it's certainly unsightly. It's what makes us overweight.

There are a number of different tables that give recommended weight ranges adjusted to height (one is included on the next page). These charts aren't of much value except to show the wide range of human variation. They don't take into consideration such individual differences as body composition (muscle weighs more than fat), skeletal size, and body type (ectomorph, mesomorph, or endomorph), all of which have an influence on weight.

The charts give arbitrary numbers and should be used only with that fact in mind, but, with or without a chart, you can tell if you're overweight. Subjectively, you know if you feel overweight and you can confirm your worst fears by looking at yourself in the mirror. Objectively, you can tell if your clothes are getting too tight and you can use the scale. If you fall outside the upper ranges of any of the height-weight charts, you are overweight.

If you are 20 percent above the recommended weight on the charts, you are probably not just overweight, but obese, a dreaded word in our society. No matter how little your food intake exceeds your energy output, you're going to put on weight. When this imbalance goes on for a time, you get overweight; if it continues, you get badly overweight; and finally, if you don't put a stop to it, you become obese.

Recommended Weight in Relation to Height *

| HEIGHT | | MEN | | WOMEN | |
FEET	INCHES	AVE.	RANGE	AVE.	RANGE
4	10	—	—	102	92-119
4	11	—	—	104	94-122
5	0	—	—	107	96-125
5	1	—	—	110	99-128
5	2	123	112-141	113	102-131
5	3	127	115-144	116	105-134
5	4	130	118-148	120	108-136
5	5	133	121-152	123	111-142
5	6	136	124-156	128	114-146
5	7	140	128-161	132	118-150
5	8	145	132-166	136	122-154
5	9	149	136-170	140	126-158
5	10	153	140-174	144	130-163
5	11	158	144-179	148	134-168
6	0	162	148-184	152	138-173
6	1	166	152-189	—	—
6	2	171	156-194	—	—
6	3	176	160-199	—	—
6	4	181	164-204	—	—

* From a table developed by the Metropolitan Life Insurance Co.

There is evidence to indicate that obesity can also result from too little physical activity as well as just overeating. One study, using pedometers, showed that nonobese subjects were twice as active as those who were obese. And factors such as heredity, body type, stress, and anxiety can also be causes of overweight and eventual obesity.

No matter the causes, if you are heavier than your "ideal" weight (usually your weight at age twenty), you are overweight. If you are 20 percent above that weight you are obese, unless you're very muscular; and if you're 25 percent over, you are subjecting yourself to potential health problems, not the least of which is heart disease.

If you can't remember your weight at twenty (or if you were

overweight then), and you can't honestly tell by looking in the mirror, then the "pinch test" is a good measure of fatness. The fat deposits under the skin quite accurately reflect the total fat stored throughout the body.

One of the best places to pinch is the back of the arm right behind the bicep. It's a little hard to take this measurement by yourself so you may want to ask a friend to help.

With your arm hanging straight down, take hold of the skin with your thumb and forefinger at the midpoint between the elbow and the shoulder. Pull the pinched area away from the muscle. The fat will pull away with skin. If you're a man under thirty the layer of fat and skin pinched away should measure less than 6/10 of an inch; for a woman, less than 1.1 inches. If you're a man over thirty, the fold should be less than 9/10 of an inch and for a woman, less than 1.25 inches. If the measurement is greater than it should be, you can consider yourself overweight, corpulent, quite plump, fat, or obese. But don't let this scare you. It's something you need to know and it's one of the reasons you're reading this book.

Body Composition

Our bodies are more than "a hank of hair and a piece of bone," as the song says. In fact, relatively, there is very little bone and even less hair. About 60 percent of body weight in men and 50 percent in women is water. Men have about 12 percent body fat on the average and women about 25 percent. The rest of the body (about 25 percent) is muscle, bone, blood, tissues, and organs, or "lean body mass."

Muscle is heavier than fat and contains much more water (about 70 percent compared to 15 percent). Since fat contains little water, the percent of total water in an obese person is lower than in a nonobese person. The relation between total water and fat-free body weight (lean body mass) should remain constant, so when you're overweight, body composition is distorted.

A combination of diet and exercise will result in the loss of fat (a large proportion of body weight), the addition of muscle, and is a very effective method of restoring the body's composition and shape.

Intensive physical training using the Mentzer Method will increase muscle mass and reduce the body's fat content. How? First, dynamic exercise with weights increases skeletal-muscle size and this muscle displaces fatty tissue throughout the body. Second, the Mentzer Method increases the capacity of the body's oxygen-transporting system through the cardiovascular training effect attained by the intensity of the exercise routine. It is a physiological fact that the greater the ability of the system to utilize oxygen, the greater the ability to use fat as fuel. Training increases the oxygen supply to the muscle cells so that exercise is largely performed aerobically with less lactic acid build-up. A low oxygen supply to the working muscle limits the usable fuel to carbohydrates. The less fit person produces more lactic acid which inhibits the use of fat as fuel.

Conscientious weight control, along with exercise, also serves to maintain the correct balance of water and fat to muscle, bone, and other tissues.

Diet for the Athlete

I have a friend, a competitive bodybuilder, who is so brainwashed by the health-food industry that he downs a special protein drink every two hours every day. If he doesn't have this glass of magic elixir he actually gets a headache and within a couple of days his ability to lift weights decreases because he believes he's losing the protein his muscles require for strength and growth.

Athletes have to be the worst offenders when it comes to believing in the magic power of foods and diet. The magic food or superpill may result in exceptional performance, provided, of course, that the athlete's diet is adequate in every other way. In other words, if you're not eating right, nothing will help, and even if you are eating well, the special items are only placebos. The effects are in your head, not your body.

Of course this is nothing new. Athletes have been fanatics for centuries. The first recorded attempt to influence performance through diet occurred in Greece more than 2,500 years ago. Two athletes switched from the basic vegetarian diet of the time to a meat diet, thinking that something in the meat would replace the suspected loss of muscle during heavy workouts. Just like my friend. Yet all the research done in this field is summed up by nutritionist Jean Mayer: "The concept that any well-balanced diet is all that athletes actually require for peak performance has not been superseded."

Even for competitive athletes there is no substitute for a well-balanced diet. Immediately before competition some athletes tend to eat more, but the increased energy expenditure in preparing for the events more than offsets the increased energy consumption. Research also has shown that greatly reduced or greatly increased protein consumption has no effect whatever on performance.

This all makes good sense and yet I know with certainty that my argument falls on deaf ears when it comes to athletes. So, just remember a well-balanced diet can provide you with everything you need and if you want to lose weight, 3,500 is the number to remember.

Chapter 7

Mind and Body

The goal of the Mentzer Method is total fitness. To me, fitness is more than just physical. Skeletal-muscle strength, cardiovascular ability, endurance, flexibility, and proper nutrition are all key elements in the fitness picture, but one additional factor—mental well-being—plays a major role in *total* fitness.

The poet W. H. Auden labeled our times "The Age of Anxiety," and, Zen Master Shunryu Suzuki, after observing contemporary life in the United States, said, "If you become too excited, your mind becomes rough and ragged. This is not good. If possible, try to be always calm and joyful and keep yourself from excitement."

Why are Americans anxious, tense, excited, rough, and ragged? Is it because of the great range of possibilities and choices in our lives, as philosopher Soren Kierkegaard says? Or is it our inability to discharge our physical and biological energies as Wilhelm Reich proposes? It's no doubt a combination of these and many other elements, but I think that Reich is close to the mark. The quantum increase in our collective anxiety corresponds very closely to the developments in science and technology that have virtually eliminated manual labor from our lives, labor that provided the basic physical release of our bottled-up psychic energy. This seems to be more than mere coincidence.

The concept of mind-body relationships is thousands of years

75

old. The Greeks idealized the healthy mind housed in the healthy body. Rene Descartes, the rationalist philosopher, proclaimed the doctrine of mind-body dichotomy in the seventeenth century. More recently, research has shown that physical fitness has psychological implications. Bruce Ogilvie, a psychologist at San Diego State College, has tested a cross section of athletes and found them to be in an exceptional state of mental health. Other psychosomatic studies indicate that physical changes result from psychological states.

Reich detailed the physical malfunctions that he felt resulted from chronic anxiety. He included hypertension, muscular rheumatism, emphysema, peptic ulcers, bronchial asthma, and some blood diseases in his list of anxiety-produced physical ailments. Dr. Hans Selye's research on stress in the 1930s resulted in very similar conclusions. Selye added heart attacks, migraine headaches, pains in the neck, alcoholism, and obesity to Reich's inventory, saying, "These and many other diseases are not the direct results of any pathogen but of our defective bodily or mental reactions to the stressors encountered in daily life."

Physiologist Per-Olof Astrand agrees with both Reich and Selye and feels it is also logical to assume (though the scientific evidence is incomplete) that the reverse is also true, that psychological changes result from physical changes.

It's not surprising then that a vast majority of respondents to the Perrier Fitness Study, those people who exercise and participate regularly in sports, said they feel better in general, are less tense, sleep better, and are better able to cope with life's pressures.

The Industrial Revolution and the incredible scientific advances in the last twenty-five years have freed us from the bonds of physical toil, given us abundant leisure time for pure enjoyment, and at the same time we seem to have been thrown into a state of deteriorating health that finds its mental expression in tension and anxiety and its physical expression in ulcers, high blood pressure, and heart attacks.

Stress and anxiety are big in America—big health problems and big business. Psychiatry is a growth industry, pharmaceutical houses pump out a glossary of stimulants and depressants designed to relieve a wide range of minor mental problems, and to watch television is to be bombarded by scores of advertisements for nonprescription products for headache, upset stomach, insomnia, and screaming children, or all of the aforementioned.

As a group, Americans seem extremely conscious, even proud, of the level of tension and stress in their daily lives. Stress is a badge of honor that symbolizes our status in society, the significance of our jobs, and the energy we put into "making it" and "making every minute count." It sometimes seems as if our importance as individuals is based on the amount of stress and anxiety we experience (or imagine we experience) during the course of the day.

Yet with all this emphasis on tension and stress, few of us know what stress is, its function, its effects, its importance, or what to do about it.

Thirty years ago, Hans Selye, the medical pioneer in this field, defined stress as "the nonspecific response of the body to any demand." Selye called the body's reaction to stress the "General Adaptation Syndrome" or G.A.S., a three-stage response that begins with an alarm reaction, followed by a stage of resistance, and finally by a state of exhaustion in which the body no longer can, or no longer needs to, resist. Stress causes internal chemical changes including the release of adrenaline, as well as physical reactions such as faster heart rate, increases in reflex speed and the thought processes, and muscular tension.

Under stress, either emotional or physical, we often get nervous and irritable, we overeat or don't eat at all, we drink too much alcohol, smoke more, have nervous breakdowns, even suffer heart attacks.

But stress isn't only the symptomatic reactions made so popular by the advertisements for pain relievers. It can be caused by a broken leg, a passionate kiss, intense exercise, or a physically dangerous situation. Pleasure and success, failure and disease all produce considerable stress. The fact is, everyone is under some degree of stress at all times. It is an unavoidable fact of life. In short, stress is the sum total of the wear and tear on the body over a lifetime. Its impact, physically and emotionally, depends on how we adapt to it and what we do to dissipate it. If Selye is right, we all have a limited amount of adaptation energy to compensate for the effects of stress, so it only makes sense that we use this adaptation energy as economically and efficiently as possible.

Today we are constantly challenged by situations that simulate the G.A.S. Traffic on the freeway, fear of crime, and competition on the job continually throw the G.A.S. apparatus into high gear. But unlike our immediate ancestors, we don't have the built-in outlets for our physical energies. The automobile has taken away the need to walk and everything from the vacuum cleaner to the food processor has served to take the physical strain out of living. There are no ready outlets for our pent-up emotions and aggressions. As a result there is ample evidence of tension everywhere around us, and spiraling death and disability rates from what Selye calls "the diseases of civilization."

Reich was' one of the first psychotherapists to take a physical approach to the mind-body question. In the 1930s he broke from the "talk therapy" of his mentor Freud and pursued the problem on a more biological level. Reich theorized he couldn't work on the psyche without working on the soma, or body, as well. His work led to the formulation of a therapy he called "orgonomy," which involved the freeing of dammed-up biological energy through the application of pressure to certain "holding points" in the muscles. He also used a series of exotic exercises to accomplish the same end. Reich discovered the existence of a continuous bioelectric field he called the "orgone," a field of energy running from the center to the periphery of the body. "Physic health," Reich said, "is characterized by the alternation between unpleasurable struggle and happiness, error and truth, deviation and rectification, rational hate and rational love; in short by being fully alive in all situations of life." He felt that such states of being as pleasure and anxiety, seemingly antithetical, actually stem from the same energy source.

Pleasure, Reich felt, is the subjective sensation of expansion, the flow of the orgone energy from the center of the body to the periphery, while anxiety resulted from the stoppage of this energy flow by what he called "armoring," which is really muscular tension. Reich maintained that unless our physical and biological energies are discharged they will eventually consume us. This discharge can be sexual, through the orgasm, Reich says, or purely physical, through exercise. Iron-pumping star Arnold Schwarzenegger combines both when he compares the pleasurable feelings of the muscle "pump" that comes from repeated muscular contractions in weight training to the equally pleasurable feelings of the orgasm.

Several years ago, I underwent a period of Reichian therapy and my observations during that time validated for me Reich's notions about energy flow. After each weekly session of special manipulations and exercises, I left the doctor's office free of even the slightest trace of muscular tension and anxiety. This feeling usually lasted for several days before wearing off.

There are other therapeutic approaches in use today that recognize the need to relieve a person's dammed-up energies. Alexander Lowen, the originator of bioenergetics, has his patients perform vigorous exercises to promote the free flow and release of their physical (and therefore emotional) anxieties. Ida Rolf and others have also developed therapies that include the manipulation of muscles as an integral part of each session.

During the development of the Mentzer Method of high-intensity exercise I've been able to document further the sensation of relief from muscular tension that follows each workout. My gym sessions actually serve to keep me on an even emotional keel. But this shouldn't be surprising. Muscles perform their work and use energy by contracting. The more intense the exercise, the more energy used, thus completely dissipating the excess energy build-up that is psychologically and sometimes physically experienced as tension.

I'm not saying that intense physical exercise attacks the causes of tension which may be rooted in the individual's personality, only that exercise can serve to rob anxiety of its fuel and keep it manageable. Exercise itself is a direct form of stress that evokes the same bodily response (G.A.S.) as stressful emotional experiences. The more intense the stressful situation, the more intense is the nature of the body's response. The Mentzer Method is unique in that the level of stress can be controlled through the structure of the exercises and can be increased or lowered as the body's needs dictate.

Next time you come home from work with a stiff neck, instead of taking an aspirin or downing a martini, try fifteen or twenty shoulder shrugs with a moderate weight on the bar. Shrugs act directly on the trapezius muscle at the base of the neck and relieve tension build-up. Try twenty or so sit-ups the next time you have a nervous stomach. Sit-ups work the entire abdominal area to free the energy and relieve anxiety.

I think intensive exercise is an antidote to stress and will help ward off "the diseases of civilization." The exercises in this book serve to increase the body's stress tolerance, which in turn reduces the drain on the reserves of adaptation energy. In short, the Mentzer Method enhances mental health as well as physical health. A combination that adds up to *total* fitness.

PART II

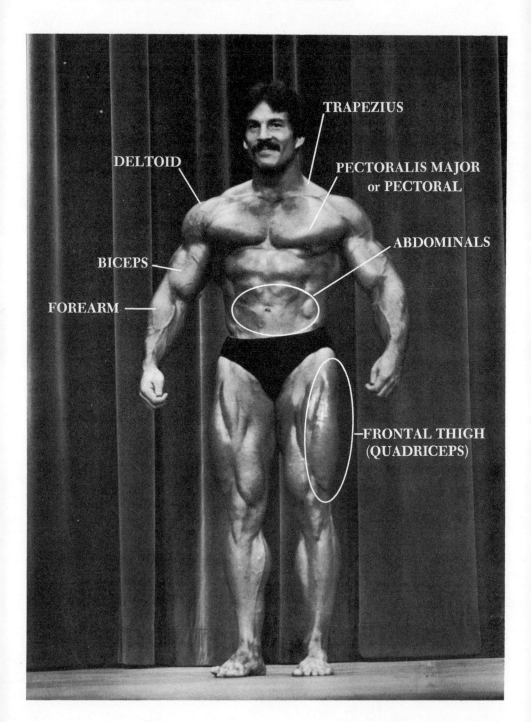

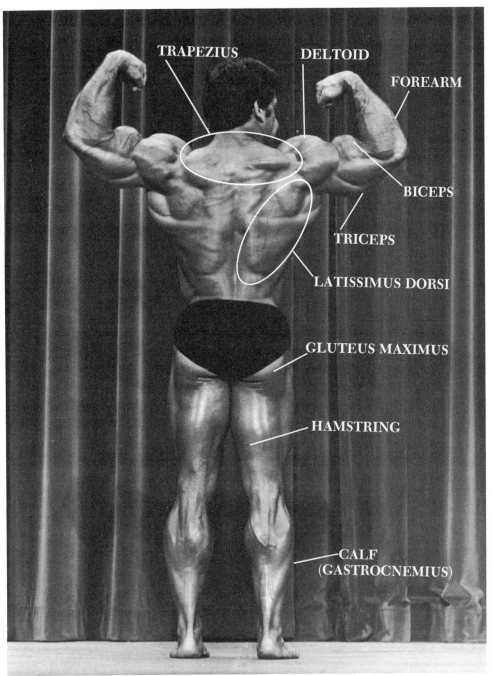

Chapter 1

What the Mentzer Method
Can Do for You

I've made hundreds of personal apperances in this country and abroad in the last few years and I've talked with thousands of people about physical fitness, weight training, diet, and nutrition. After each workshop or seminar I answer questions and the question I'm asked most is, "Will your program work for me?"

The answer is an unequivocal, "Yes." I don't care if you're five or even 150 pounds overweight, whether you're short or tall, male or female, old or young, weak or strong, in shape or out. The Mentzer Method will work for you. It will work because it's based on a solid scientific foundation, because it's sound physiologically and nutritionally.

I fully realize that most of you have tried the fads and the gimmicks, vitamins and food supplements, crash diets, and exercise machines. I know you're looking for a rational, well-researched approach to exercise and diet that will keep your heart healthy and your body in shape for a lifetime. The Mentzer Method will help you achieve that goal. If I didn't feel so strongly that weight training is the single most effective type of exercise for total fitness, I wouldn't have bothered to write this book.

Here, once more, is what the Mentzer Method will do for you if you follow it faithfully and incorporate its principles into your lifestyle.

The Mentzer Method will:

—Build skeletal-muscle strength
—Increase cardiovascular efficiency
—Increase joint mobility and overall flexibility
—Decrease mental stress
—Help you lose weight and keep it off
—Improve your overall physical appearance
—Improve your self-image
—Increase your body consciousness
—Help prevent heart disease, ulcers, nervous disorders, and other stress-related diseases.

Here's why the Mentzer Method works. Most physiologists now agree that physical fitness is determined by three measurements: 1) Your capacity for energy output (cardiovascular efficiency); 2) Muscular strength and coordination; and 3) The mobility of your joints. A good training program will meet these three criteria.

The Mentzer Method, by stimulating a cardiovascular training effect, increases your capacity for energy output (energy output is also a critical factor in weight control). Through dynamic exercise the Mentzer Method improves your muscular strength and coordination. By working the muscles through a full range of motion the Mentzer Method increases joint mobility.

Here's how it works. Bursts of intense activity (working with weights) lasting but for a few seconds can develop muscular strength, strengthen tendons and ligaments, and improve flexibility. These bursts of activity maintained over a period of just one minute help develop anaerobic power, and when this exercise lasts for three to five minutes it develops aerobic power. And, the weight-training routines described here, when sustained for thirty minutes, serve to further develop the oxygen-transporting system and increase endurance.

No other form of exercise can provide all of these measurements of physical fitness. This is what makes the Mentzer Method so unique.

And there is a plus in the Mentzer Method. The intense physical activity of weight training actually relieves muscular tension and releases nervous energy, thus reducing stress and effectively removing a potential cause of stress-related physical disorders.

Your complete health prescription can be filled by the Mentzer Method. It is total.

Let's work together now to achieve the level of fitness—total fitness—we've been talking about. If you follow this program closely, the results will come so quickly you'll be amazed. But please remember that there are no magic exercises. To be effective, physical training requires work and sweat. On the other hand, it doesn't have to be unpleasant. I think you'll find the Mentzer Method surprisingly pleasant and I know you'll find it rewarding.

About the Exercises

The exercises described in the following sections are standard weight-resistance exercises, and have been used by athletes all over the world since the invention of the plate-loading barbell. As you become familiar with the various exercises you'll find yourself liking some more than others. That's natural. For example, I really like the squat. Most people hate squats because of the exertion involved. And arm exercises, the favorite of most people, don't excite me at all.

Likes and dislikes aside, it's very important to follow the exercise sequences as they are listed. The exercises were selected and arranged to provide all the skeletal muscles with equal work loads, to minimize localized fatigue, and to keep the pulse rate elevated. This balanced work load will prevent the development of any weak muscular links in the body.

It's important, for example, that you develop leg strength in the hamstrings (located in the back of the thighs) which lower the knee, and at the same time in the massive frontal muscle in the thigh which raises the knee. Athletes such as football and tennis players often suffer hamstring pulls because they have developed great strength in their frontal thigh muscles but have neglected the hamstrings. Muscles work in teams of opposing muscle, and the balance is delicate. The stronger of two opposing muscles can dominate the weaker and cause severe damage to tendons and other fibers. The frontal thigh generates tremendous force when engaged in an explosive effort such as charging out of the backfield or sprinting after a tennis ball. Weak links can be disastrous.

Also bear in mind that the underlying goal of the Mentzer Method is total fitness—strengthening the cardiovascular system as well as toning up and increasing muscular strength. To simplify matters the exercise descriptions are written for those who want the cardiovascular effect. This means relatively light weights and more repetitions of each dynamic movement. If you want to use heavier weights to test your strength, fine, but remember that kind of work is specifically for skeletal-muscle development and gives your cardiovascular system very little stimulation. If you perform these resistance exercises at a rapid pace with light to moderate weights and a high number of repetitions, you'll increase your cardiovascular strength and at the same time enhance your skeletal-muscle strength and tone, and you will be on your way to achieving *Total Fitness*.

About Motivation

Motivation may be the key element, and the most underrated, in any exercise or diet program. It's what makes people take action and pursue specific goals and objectives. And it may be the most important factor in successfully achieving those goals and objectives.

I think I'm highly motivated and yet there are some days when I'd love to just lie on the beach sipping lemonade rather than work out and count my calories. It's hard to keep your eye on the target even when you're a professional athlete. I can only tell you that the price of improvement is as much mental as physical.

Charles Atlas was a master of motivation. "I can make you a new man in only fifteen minutes a day if you enroll now for my Great Dynamic-Tension Course," he said. He also promised to "quickly" help us achieve a "husky body that men will respect and women admire." He certainly pressed all the right buttons: new man, fifteen minutes a day, dynamic, quick, husky, respect, admiration.

Atlas knew forty years ago that a body at rest tends to remain at rest, and his motivational message obviously got tens of thousands of bodies to move at least as far as the mailbox. For most people, it ended right there.

If Atlas was among the first to make extravagant claims about self-improvement, he was only a harmless harbinger of things to come. Today we're inundated with all kinds of wild weight-training and exercise programs, diet plans, health food claims, and self-awareness and self-help programs that are just that—wild.

In the short run, you can be temporarily motivated, even duped, but deep down you know that nothing can make you a new person in fifteen minutes a day, no diet can help you lose fourteen pounds in fourteen days and keep it off, no self-awareness workshop can make you feel good about yourself in one weekend. It's all just a hype. There are no miracles. But the lure is still there and what makes people continually take the bait is the fact that most diets work for a little while, most bodybuilding programs build a little bicep, and we all feel good about ourselves for a few days after a self-awareness marathon. We quickly forget that these improvements, often very expensive, are only temporary. What Atlas and Atkins and Erhard and all the rest fail to tell us is that instant gratification isn't enough.

What's needed is a long-term commitment. And you must be strongly motivated to make that commitment. It must be made with realistic goals in mind.

Serious bodybuilders often ask me the best and fastest way to gain muscle. They expect me to say, "Do it my way and you'll gain a pound of solid muscle a week." The truth is there is no fast way to gain muscle just as there is no fast way to lose weight. It's exactly the same kind of thinking that leads runners to start dreaming of the marathon before they've run the first mile. People just love to dream when it comes to physical fitness.

It is this type of wishful thinking that is primarily responsible for the failure of so many people who just want to improve their appearance and health by toning up and losing a little fat. Look at it this way. It probably took five, ten, or even fifteen years of inactivity and a sedentary lifestyle for you to get out of shape, and though it won't take nearly that long to get back into good shape, it won't happen overnight either.

It's important to recognize that losing body fat (not just weight, which can come off quickly in loss of body fluid), like gaining muscle, is a slow process. The body stores fat more or less uniformly, though it tends to accumulate more readily in the stomach, thighs, and hips, and we have absolutely no control over this storage process. That's why spot reducing is a myth perpetuated by commercial interests selling a variety of vibrating machines, heat belts, sweat suits, and all those other incredible appliances. These devices may shake the daylights out of you or make you sweat, but you can't shake or sweat fat away. The only reduction you can expect from spot-reducing gimmicks is a reduction in your bank account.

The time element is so important to motivation that I want to reemphasize it. It takes time to accumulate fat and it takes time to lose it. It takes time to lose muscle and it takes time to get it back. Give yourself time. Be patient. Be realistic.

Whether your goal is to be the best-built man or woman of all time or just to tone up and trim down so you look good in the mirror, success can be achieved and maintained only if you develop a lifelong commitment to exercise and sensible diet. If this sounds too hard (and I don't think it does), then you're probably reading the wrong book. But I want to hammer home the point that exercise doesn't have to be unpleasant, it doesn't have to be a chore. In fact, it should be extremely pleasant, enjoyable, and rewarding. It has to be for you to keep at it. And weight training offers the easiest means of assessing the physical rewards of exercise: the tape measure, the mirror, and the scale. You can actually see, feel, and document your progress. There is no better motivation.

My program comes with no guarantee, but I can promise you that you can dramatically improve your appearance and your mental outlook while increasing your total level of physical fitness if you properly apply the basic exercise and weight-control principles of the Mentzer Method. It will surprise you. It will quickly become part of an enjoyable and rewarding lifestyle and it will motivate you to further achievements.

Chapter 2

A Little Explanation

Here are a few points to keep in mind before you actually bend over and pick up that first barbell or dumbbell.

See Your Doctor

I strongly advise you to see your doctor before embarking on this total fitness program. Even if you feel fit or if you've been training for some time, it's still prudent to get a medical opinion on your general state of health. If you're past thirty, a thorough physical examination is a must and a stress electrocardiogram is a good idea.

If you have high blood pressure, if you're overweight, if you have a known heart condition, or a family history of heart problems, take special note of the following: Blood pressure during arm work (and much of this program demands arm work) is higher than in leg work. The heart rate is therefore higher and this puts a heavier load on the heart's pumping capacity. Dynamic exercise of the skeletal muscles increases the muscle pump. This is very effective in getting the blood to the heart and it produces an immediate increase in cardiac output. The normal heart can pump all the blood it receives but the abnormal heart cannot. Thus, heavy arm-work can be dangerous for people with heart problems, completely untrained people, and older people. *Don't start this program if you have any doubts.*

Interestingly, isometric exercises are an even greater danger because they result in a far higher blood pressure level than dynamic work. This can be extremely dangerous to a person with any kind of heart condition.

It's also important to be on the lookout for physical symptoms after you begin exercising. If you have chest pains, feel dizzy, if your heart rate stays high, stop exercising and go back to the doctor for another look.

It's most important to be careful. Use your common sense. See a doctor and get an OK before you start this, or any other, program.

Circuit Training

The Mentzer Method utilizes at least one venerated weight-training technique—circuit training. This procedure has stood the test of time and it works. Circuit training simply means a series of activities performed one after the other and then repeated at the end of the last activity in the series. By experimenting, the weight trainer can perform the various exercises at maximal exertion and determine the number of repetitions and weight for each exercise. The advantage to this type of training is that each person can adjust the program to meet his or her fitness level. Improvement can be easily measured by recording the weight used and the time required for the exercises. Retesting after a predetermined time period will clearly show the changes. More repetitions, heavier weights, and shorter times all indicate progress and help to maintain motivation.

Overload

Skeletal and heart muscles grow when they are stimulated by exercise. But the exercise, to be effective, must expose the body to stress of sufficient intensity to produce an improvement in whatever functions are being trained. To achieve that level of intensity the body has to be exposed to an "overload," a level of stress that is greater than normal. Obviously, the training load is relative to the fitness level of the individual.

The more fit a person is, the more intense the exercise must be to improve on the level of fitness. Therefore, as you improve and become more fit, you'll have to increase the intensity of your training. When the body adapts to a given load, the training intensity has to be increased to achieve further improvement. The scientific reason for the need for overload training for improvement isn't completely known but it is accepted as fact by most physiologists.

Fatigue

When Roger Bannister broke the four-minute barrier in the mile run more than twenty-five years ago, he collapsed as he crossed the finish line. He was completely fatigued and didn't recover for some time. His fatigue was obviously extreme.

There are two causes of fatigue: a drop in the level of blood sugar in the body, and the accumulation of lactic acid in muscles that have been depleted of oxygen through intense work. Though a problem in most other intense-exercise programs, neither of these factors should cause difficulty in my program of weight training. For one thing you can easily replenish your supply of blood sugar by taking liquids as necessary, and second, the workout sessions are short enough to prevent any oxygen debt or lactic acid build-up.

Soreness

Physiologists still haven't discovered the exact causes of muscle soreness but everyone knows the pain of sore, overexercised muscles. When an untrained person, or a trained person for that matter, exercises vigorously, the muscles stiffen and harden and become sore. The first symptoms usually appear about twelve hours after exercising, the pain becomes more severe the next day, then gradually fades away after three or four days. I vividly remember a number of incidents in my training career when, in a fit of enthusiasm, I'd embark on a vigorous, high-intensity routine after a lay-off. Even a week off will do it. One incident in particular comes to mind. My high school graduation gift from my father was a trip to Florida. On my second day in Tampa

I visited one of the better-known bodybuilding gyms and was introduced to Jim Haslop, then Mr. America, who was training there. Out of the blue he asked me if I wanted to train my legs with him. Though I hadn't trained in a week, I jumped at the rare opportunity to work out with a Mr. America. Determined to keep pace with Haslop, I did about twenty sets of very heavy toe raises that day and I remember leaving the gym beaming with pride at having matched Mr. America in a workout. The next day I wasn't beaming. My calves were so sore from the toe raises that for four days I couldn't get out of bed. For four days it was so bad I actually had to crawl to the bathroom.

Soreness is probably caused by tiny injuries to the connective tissue in the muscles and at points where the muscles attach to the tendons. It's the repair of this damaged tissue that results in a stronger muscle, much less likely to get sore in the future even with more severe exercise. It's actually a positive result but unless you're a masochist you'll want to avoid as much soreness as possible. Take heed and break in slowly.

Maintenance

As far-fetched as it may seem, within about four weeks you'll already have developed a reasonable level of fitness and strength by following the Mentzer Method. At the end of eight weeks, the improvement will be marked. But don't become complacent or self-satisfied. These gains can be lost very quickly if you stop training for even a short time. In fact, all your gains can be lost in as little as five weeks if you stop training altogether. Year-around training is a must for the cardiovascular system, but it is also important for the skeletal muscles because strength gains can also be lost with upsetting quickness.

The good news is that less effort is required to maintain a high level of fitness than to reach that level in the first place. This means hard work at first can pay off later in shorter and less frequent workouts if you prefer.

Overtraining

Overtraining is the other side of maintenance. When you begin to make those initial gains in strength and endurance, you'll find it hard to resist the urge to train more often than suggested in the hope that more work will result in faster development. Resist the urge because it doesn't pay. In the first place, it takes at least forty-eight hours to completely replace the body's depleted glycogen stores and secondly, your muscles need time to recover and rebuild. The small additional gains you can make take a disproportionate amount of work and are simply not worth it.

Breathing

Most books on exercise spend an awful lot of time trying to explain in exhaustive and confusing detail something that comes naturally. They tell you when to breathe and how much and when to stop. It can get to the point where you're nearly immobilized by instructions. Actually, it's when you do the most thinking about it that you make mistakes. Like the centipede which, when asked how it was able to walk on so many legs, thought about it, tried to move, and fell over.

As the body is subjected to increased muscular activity there is a vastly increased demand for oxygen by all the tissues, especially muscle tissue. To meet this need it's necessary to breath harder and faster. As long as the requirement for oxygen is met, either through aerobic or anaerobic processes, the exercise can continue. In the first two minutes of work, anaerobic power is the most important factor but at about two minutes the ratio is 50 percent anaerobic-50 percent aerobic and after two minutes aerobic power dominates. This means that after only a couple of minutes your body is making full use of the oxygen it's taking in.

The Mentzer Method makes it possible to control the intensity of effort and remain in the aerobic zone for twelve to fifteen minutes of continuous activity. If you can't sustain a workout for that long because of breathing problems, then the intensity of the exercise is too high for you. If this happens you won't be benefiting your cardiovascular system or your muscles either.

As you follow the exercises in this book, try to establish a controlled rhythm in your breathing. Inhale when lifting or pressing a weight and exhale when you lower it. This rhythm will become natural very quickly.

The most important thing to remember is *never hold your breath while lifting*. Exerting yourself, especially with your arms, while holding your breath prevents the air from leaving your lungs and radically increases the pressure of the blood which is being pumped to the heart and brain, creating a greater pressure within the chest cavity.

Proper rhythmic breathing will allow you to work out with less fatigue because it facilitates oxygen transport.

Equipment

One of the most attractive features of this fitness program is that it can be performed in a relatively confined space—your bedroom or garage or back porch—in any kind of weather, and with a minimum investment in equipment. All you really need is a plate-loading barbell set that allows you to adjust the poundage, and a pair of dumbbell handles. These usually come in one package and sell for about $30. You can also make use of a watch or clock with a sweep second hand for checking your pulse rate, and later you may want to add a bench for pressing and a few other exercises (about $30 at most sporting goods stores). Used properly, barbells produce very good results but remember, for $60 we're not talking about equipping a luxury health spa. If you want that kind of equipment, it is available, but you will have to pay a good bit for it.

Gyms—Health Clubs

Many people enjoy exercising more, and even find it easier, if other people are involved. If you're one of those people it might pay to invest in a gym or health-club membership. Most cities have a variety of facilities ranging from serious bodybuilding gyms (some of which resemble dungeons) to the very posh, luxury spas with everything from deep-pile carpet to whirlpool baths and Swedish saunas. Most facilities have more than enough equipment for you to get started on this program so you'll want to do a little shopping around to see which offers the best in price, atmosphere, and supervision.

If I was joining a club, I'd think seriously about one of the Nautilus Fitness Centers. Most Nautilus centers are staffed with trained personnel who have a basic understanding of the essentials of exercise physiology. They have at their disposal the latest in sophisticated exercise equipment and they are committed to helping their clients improve. They emphasize the need for effort and dedication, unlike the sugar coating you get at some of the better known and more expensive health spas.

If you think the gym atmosphere is right for you, go to it.

Pulse Monitoring

Remember that the basic requirement for increasing cardiovascular fitness is exercise that will elevate your pulse rate to your age-adjusted level (see chart on page 98) and keep it there for twelve to fifteen minutes. If you have read this far, you've probably had a physical examination and, if you're past thirty, a stress electrocardiogram. From this you know how high you can raise your pulse rate without overstressing your heart.

For pulse monitoring, weight training is the ideal exercise because, unlike jogging and many other sports, you can stop at any time and get an accurate count.

There are ten spots on the body (not including the heart itself) where the pulse wave can be clearly felt and counted. The artery on the thumb side of the wrist is most often used but during exercise it is easier to use the large arteries (carotid) at the side of the neck. To find the neck artery, put your thumb on your chin, cupping the chin in the hollow between the thumb and forefinger. From that position the fingers can easily find the artery in front of the thick muscle that runs vertically in the neck. To get an accurate count you have to take it immediately after stopping your exercise because the pulse rate (and therefore the heart rate) drops very quickly. After you've found the beat, count it for ten seconds. Multiply that number by six and you'll have your pulse rate for one minute. Don't count for more than ten seconds because the rate falls too fast for accuracy.

After a few workouts you will begin to recognize your body's response when your pulse rate moves into the training level

Maximum Attainable Heart Rate and Cardiovascular Training Effect Zone *

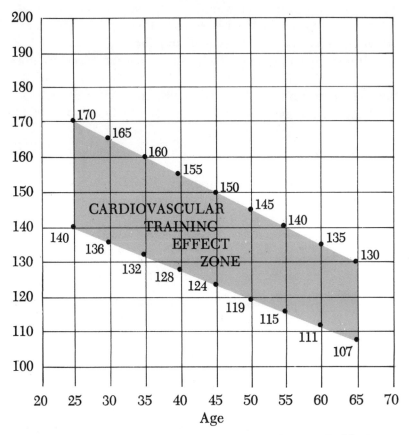

* Adapted from *Exercise Your Way to Fitness And Heart Health*, American Heart Association and President's Council on Physical Fitness and Sports, 1974.

but until then it's best to take your pulse before warming up, immediately after the sequence of exercises, and finally after you've completed your cool-down routine. If your pulse rate is still below 60 percent of your maximum during the strenuous part of your workout, you'll have to increase the intensity of your work. On the other hand, if your pulse rate is pushing 85 percent of your maximum, it's best to cut back on intensity.

I've included a sample progress chart. If you use it regularly, you'll soon see the visible evidence of your progress and this, along with the mental and physical evidence of your development, will keep your enthusiasm high.

Intensity—Duration—Frequency

These three words are fundamental to the Mentzer Method. They signify the difference between my exercise program and all the others. By intensity I don't mean furrowing your brow and giving the bar a hard look, though concentration is definitely involved. And I don't necessarily mean the use of very heavy weights though the amount of weight you use certainly affects the intensity of the exercise. By intensity I mean carrying each individual exercise to the point where you just can't do any more, where one more repetition is literally impossible. Most weight trainers refer to this ultimate limit as the point of momentary muscular failure. And by intensity I also mean moving quickly from one exercise to another, allowing very little time between each one. Training intensity has long been one of the hotly debated subjects among physical fitness professionals but most trainers, coaches, and physiologists now agree that the greater the intensity of the exercise the better. Maintenance of a high level of intensity is what results in the cardiovascular training effect.

The intensity of your workout essentially determines its duration as well. When you're working at maximum capacity, your strength and energy reserves limit the length of your workout. And that's the idea. Better results can be obtained from short sessions than from much longer sessions. It's really a question of energy cost. During heavy exercise the energy demand is high and the supply is limited. If, for example, you and a friend go bike riding on a two-mile course and you finish the course in half the time taken by your friend, you will both have used the same amount of energy but the intensity of your effort, your exercise, has been greater.

The frequency of your workouts is also determined in large measure by their intensity. The muscles and the glycogen stores both need time to replenish themselves. Three thirty-minute workouts a week will be all you can, or should try to, handle.

Exercise Performance

The Zen master says, "The most important point in practice is to have right and perfect effort . . . Become proud of your practice."

This maxim can be applied equally to weight training and exercise in general. Scientific studies have shown that barbell exercises initiated with a sudden jerk and completed rapidly apply resistance only at the beginning and the end of the movement. Slow and deliberate movements, however, apply resistance to the entire length of the muscle and are much more productive. High-speed movements also produce their own momentum which then substitutes for muscular contraction in the completion of the exercise. It's imperative that all the exercise routines that follow be performed from beginning to end in a *slow and steady fashion.* The weight should leave the starting position (usually the fully extended position) smoothly, without jerking or throwing. The same slow rhythm should be maintained throughout each movement, using muscular contraction alone as the means of movement. If you use only muscular contraction you'll be able to hold the weight in its final position or at any point in the entire range of motion for the exercise. This is because, physiologically, your ability to hold weight is greater than your ability to lift the same weight.

Lowering the weight (negative resistance) should take at least as long and maybe a little longer than raising the weight. Some exercise physiologists believe the negative motion provides a greater training effect than the positive movement. Depending on the exercise, each complete repetition should take between seven and ten seconds.

Smooth and controlled exercise performance is also an important factor in injury prevention. Lifting a moderate weight by the force of muscular contraction alone makes it almost impossible to injure a muscle or tendon. Trying to yank, jerk, or throw the same weight, however, amplifies the actual force imposed on the muscles and joints and greatly increases the risk of injury. Slow, smooth, and steady are the words to remember.

The Proper Weight

The proper weight selection for each of the exercises in this program is going to take some experimentation. You don't know how strong you are so don't jump to any conclusions. It's obvious that some of your muscles are naturally stronger than others so it will be necessary to change weights at times throughout your training session.

Choose a weight that allows for the proper performance of from twelve to fifteen repetitions of the exercise. Weights that allow for only six repetitions or so are fine for producing greater strength but remember your priority is to achieve total fitness along with skeletal-muscle tone and strength. At least twelve repetitions are necessary to sufficiently elevate the pulse and enhance cardiovascular fitness.

You'll know you've got the right amount of weight if the eleventh and twelfth repetitions require a near maximal effort. If you can easily do twelve, don't kid yourself. Put some more weight on the bar.

After a relatively short time your strength will increase and the weight that allowed only twelve repetitions will now allow twenty. When this happens, increase the weight about 10 percent and this should reduce your repetitions to twelve. Such is the nature of progressive weight training. You have to keep making it harder for yourself.

To keep your pulse rate up for twelve to fifteen minutes you're going to have to move quickly between exercises. That doesn't mean doing fast repetitions. It means the time used for changing weights and beginning the next exercise has to be kept to a minimum. As your fitness increases it will be harder to maintain your high pulse rate and at that point more intense effort on your part will be required.

Are you ready? OK. Then let's get started.

Chapter 3

Let's Get to It

Theory is one thing, practice another. It's time to put on your exercise clothes. Since all the exercise routines in this book are designed to meet the requirements of total fitness, it's necessary to get mentally and physically ready for them. I think it's important to spend at least one week (probably more) breaking in, temporarily restraining your desire to move ahead to the more intense exercises. This break-in period will also help you avoid some of the soreness and fatigue that can be expected when starting any exercise program.

The amount of time you spend breaking in depends on your current levels of fitness, but regardless of how fit you are, I recommend one full week of break-in time and up to four weeks if you have been inactive for a year or more.

I also think it's advisable to work out five days during the first week for about twenty minutes each day. The exercises are of moderate intensity so your recovery time will be quite short. If you need more than a week to get ready, stay with the five-day plan but increase your exercise time to thirty minutes a session.

These initial sessions, like all the workouts in this book, begin with a warm-up period, followed by a series of basic exercises for each body part, and conclude with a cool-down routine. During the break-in only one set of exercises for each body part will be necessary. This one set consists of twelve repetitions and in this case the twelfth should still be quite easy. Take as much time as you need, resting between exercises if necessary, and don't worry about your pulse rate. I don't want you breathing hard when you're through, but you should be pleasantly fatigued. This period also will give you the chance to perfect your form and discover how strong you are. You'll have time to experiment with different weights and practice getting them on and off the bars.

None of the exercises that follow is complicated. I've tried to describe them in the most concise and understandable language and you can use the photos as guides. The important thing is to feel comfortable, so if the directions say to stand with your feet shoulder-width apart and that doesn't feel quite right, make the necessary adjustments. The main thing in most of these exercises is that you have a solid base, a well-balanced foundation so you won't sway or topple over.

Warm-up

It's hard to overemphasize the importance of warm-up exercises in preparation for any athletic activity. They help prevent injury (more people suffer muscle pulls and tears because of insufficient warm-up than for any other reason), they improve your performance, and they get you psychologically ready for the more intense work to come. And strenuous exercise without proper warm-up can produce an abnormal heart rate.

I'm sure you've noticed that when you first begin exercising, even walking, you feel sluggish. This is because the exchange of oxygen from the blood to the tissues and muscles is being adjusted by the body to meet the new demand. As your body and muscle temperature rise this exchange is much more rapid and a steady state develops where the oxygen intake equals the oxygen requirements of the tissues. You are warming up.

I strongly recommend warm-up exercises that stretch rather than the more traditional calisthenics style because calisthenics don't do a thing for flexibility and the movements generally bear no relation to the type of exercise activity that follows. At least five minutes of warm-up is necessary and ten to fifteen minutes is better (more than fifteen minutes is relatively unproductive).

The benefits of the warm-up will be lost if you then wait more than fifteen minutes to begin exercising. Wearing slightly warmer clothing during warm-up is also helpful.

Cool-down

Don't just stop and flop. During strenuous exercise the pulse rate and blood circulation increase rapidly. It's possible to reach your maximum heart rate in as little as one minute if the exercise is heavy and it's been preceded by a sufficient warm-up period. In less heavy exercise the maximum rate is reached in roughly two to six minutes. From its resting state to a highly active state the muscle cell can increase its consumption of fuel and oxygen fifty times. This is a shock to the system, a stressful situation to which the body reacts quickly by matching oxygen intake and oxygen demand.

If you stop exercising suddenly, the heart, which has been hard at work, tends to maintain an elevated rate and continues to provide an abnormally high rate of blood circulation. This can cause dizziness or muscle cramps.

A cool-down period of moderate stretching and bending exercises will help prevent this sudden bodily change and give the heart a chance to adjust again to its normal level of activity. These cool-downs, like the warm-ups, should take from five to fifteen minutes.

Here is a one-week break-in routine that will get your body and mind ready for the more intense exercises in the next chapter.

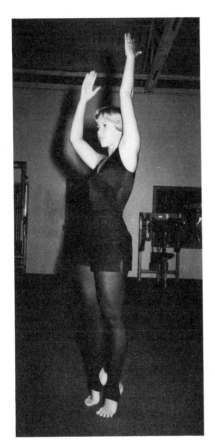
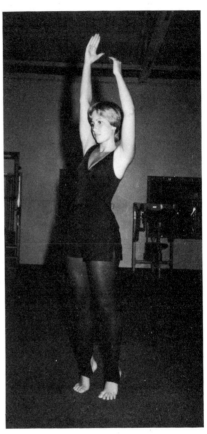

Warm-ups—Approximately Fifteen Minutes

1) Overhead Arm Stretches—Stand with your back straight and your arms stretched straight up; elbows close to the ears. Stretch your right arm as high as you can toward the ceiling. Your right shoulder and right hip will also move upward and your heels will come off the floor. Relax the right arm and let it come back to the starting position and repeat the movement with the left arm. Stretch as high as you can each time and you'll soon begin to feel the muscles in the arms, shoulders, and sides stretching and warming.

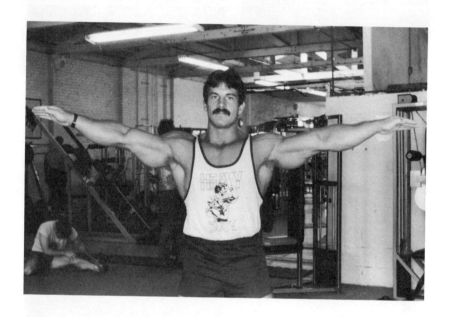

2) Arm Circles—Stand with your feet slightly spread and your arms straight out from your sides. Begin by slowly rotating both arms in small clockwise circles. Gradually enlarge the circles until they are about twelve inches in diameter. Then gradually decrease the size until you're again making small circles. Slowly stop and repeat by rotating your arms in the opposite direction. Keep your arms as straight as you can and you'll feel the movement in your upper arms and shoulders.

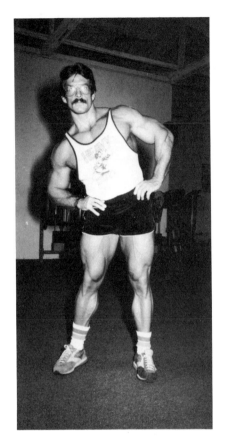

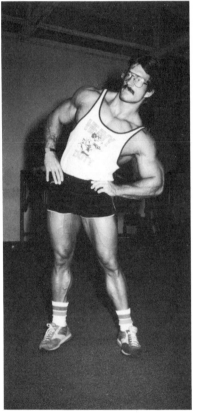

3) Side Bends—With feet about shoulder-width apart, back straight, and hands on hips, bend to the right as far as possible without moving the hips—bend at the waist. Return to the starting position and bend to the left. The muscles in the lower back and the sides will benefit from this movement.

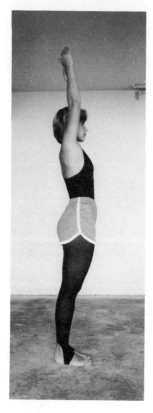

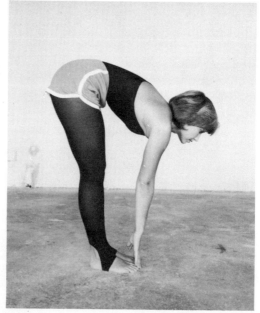

4) Toe Touches—Stand with your back straight and your feet slightly spread. Stretch your arms straight overhead with the elbows close to the ears. Now, in one motion bend over and touch your toes without bending your knees, keeping your head between your arms throughout the entire movement. Slowly return to the starting position and repeat. The stretching takes place in the back of the legs and at the waist.

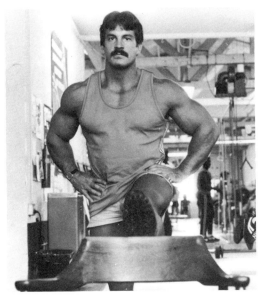

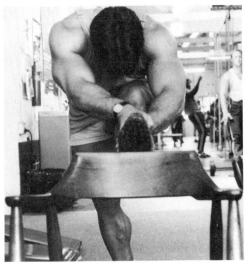

5) Leg Stretches—You'll need a low chair for this one. Plant one foot firmly on the floor and put the heel of the other foot on the back of the chair a couple of feet in front of you. Keeping both legs as straight as possible, bend forward at the waist. Try to touch the toes of the raised foot with the fingers of both hands and bring your head as close as you can to your outstretched knee; hold for a second. Repeat five times and then switch legs. This will stretch the backs of your legs from thigh to calf.

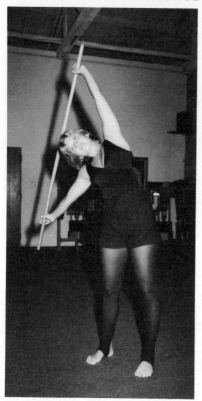
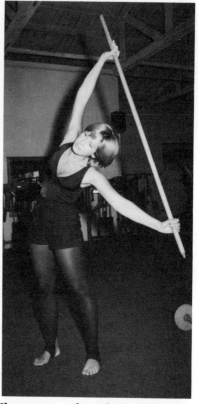

6) Body Stretch—This exercise will warm up the whole body, get the blood flowing, and get your mind off the problems of the day. Stand with your back straight, your feet about shoulder-width apart and your arms stretched full length straight over your head. I find it helpful to hold a broomstick or a five- to ten-pound dumbbell for this exercise. Now slowly bend to one side, keeping your head between your arms and your back straight. Bend as far as you can to one side without bouncing and stretch so that you can feel the muscles along the side pulling. Return to the starting position and then bend to the other side. Repeat ten times for each side. Remember to keep stretching and don't bend forward. Try not to thrust your pelvis forward but to keep the body in a straight, vertical plane.

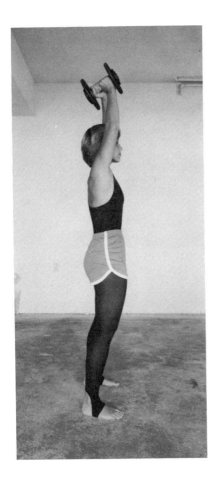

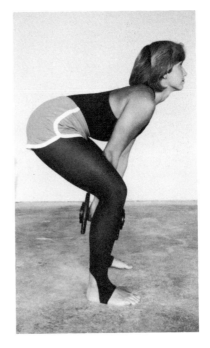

7) Tree Chopping—Stand with your legs spread apart far enough to allow your arms to swing between them. Holding a light dumbbell with both hands, raise your arms straight over your head. Now, as if you were chopping a log, bring your arms down, keeping them straight, bend at the waist, and swing the dumbbell between your legs as far as you can. You will feel the back of your legs stretch.

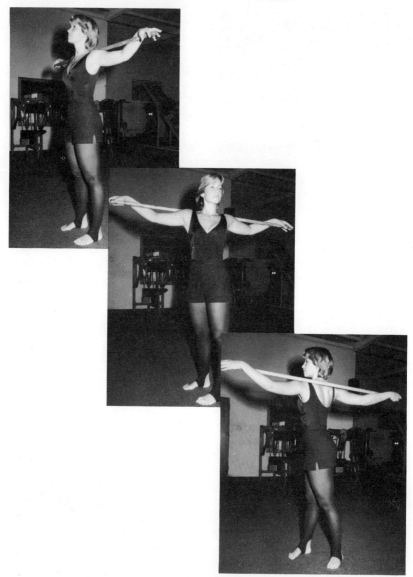

8) Twists—With your feet a little more than shoulder-width apart, place the broomstick behind your head, and hold it where it feels comfortable. Keeping the pole parallel to the floor and keeping your hips and head as straight as possible, twist your torso and swing one end of the pole as far as you can in front of you. Come back to center and swing the pole and twist your torso in the other direction.

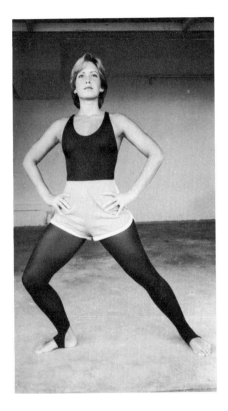
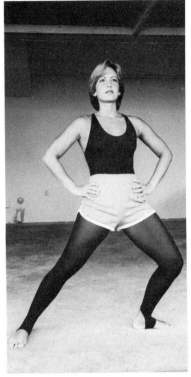

9) Side Lunges—This exercise is especially effective for warming up the legs, pelvic area, and the knees. It's done without weights. Stand erect with your feet together and your hands on your hips. Begin by stepping out to the right at about a 45-degree angle, placing the right foot firmly on the floor and keeping the left foot planted. Be sure to keep your back straight, your head up, and your hands on your hips. Return to the starting position and repeat the same movement to the left side. You should feel a good stretch in the thigh area of both legs.

There are dozens of warm-up exercises you can substitute for those suggested here and it's not a bad idea to change from time to time for the sake of variety. Just remember to combine a series of warm-ups that work the sides, back, shoulders, and legs, and put some real effort into it so they actually "warm up" all parts of the body.

Break-in Exercises—Approximately Thirty Minutes

Each of these exercises is effective for at least one body part and several of them work the whole body through the one muscle or set of muscles the exercise is primarily designed to stimulate. The large muscles will be worked first because they are strongest and take more energy to activate, but also because the large-muscle groups must be engaged to efficiently achieve a cardiovascular training effect. There is another advantage, too. The body can tolerate a longer work or exercise period when a larger mass of skeletal muscles is activated. It's more efficient and psychologically less strenuous.

Exercise No. 1—Squats

MUSCLES EXERCISED—Thighs

Comment—if I had to choose a favorite exercise, this would be the one. Squats are relatively taxing but that's what makes them so productive. In a very short time the thighs will show the effects of squats but at the same time the entire body benefits because most of the large muscles are involved.

Directions—Stand with your feet comfortably apart, adjusting your position until you feel strong and stable. Bend over, flexing the knees, and grasp the bar with an overhand (palms down) grip. Your hands should be slightly more than shoulder-width apart. Raise the bar and place it behind the head so that it rests across the shoulders, a little below the neck. Keeping your back and head straight, "squat" by lowering yourself slowly until your thighs are nearly parallel with the floor. Make sure your feet are flat on the floor at all times. Then, without bouncing out of the bottom position, slowly raise yourself back to the starting position. Repeat twelve times.

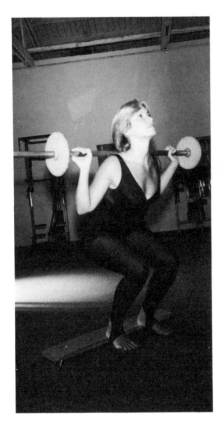
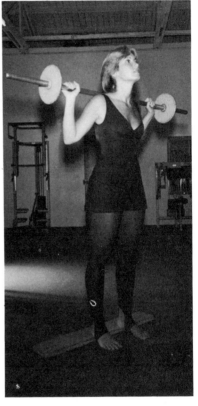

Reminder—Pay close attention to your style. Be careful not to let your thighs go below parallel with the floor because the knees can become hyperextended. A bounce at the bottom only makes it worse for the knees and the lower back.

Hint—Keep your eyes on the point where the ceiling meets the wall. This will force you to hold your head up and keep your back straight. You may want to put a board under your heels for added balance.

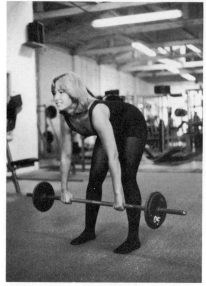

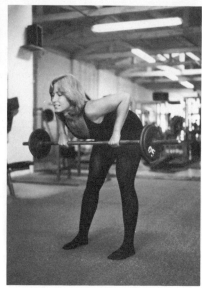

Exercise No. 2—Barbell Rows

MUSCLES EXERCISED—Back

Comment—This is perhaps the best exercise for the back. It works the entire shoulder area as well as the fine muscles of the upper back and the broad latissimus dorsi muscles in the clavicles (the collarbones).

Directions—Spread your feet comfortably apart, bend over at the waist, knees slightly bent, head up. Grasp the bar in an over-handed grip with the hands about shoulder-width apart. Keeping your back as nearly parallel with the floor as possible, pull the barbell to your chest and lower it slowly back until it almost touches the floor. Repeat twelve times.

Hint—You will be able to handle a lot of weight in this exercise and your strength will increase quickly, so if you find yourself capable of doing twenty repetitions in a couple of weeks, be sure to increase the weight and get yourself back to a dozen.

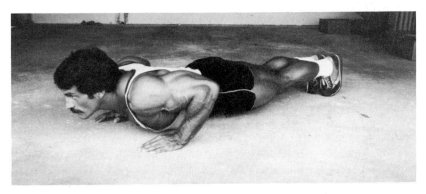

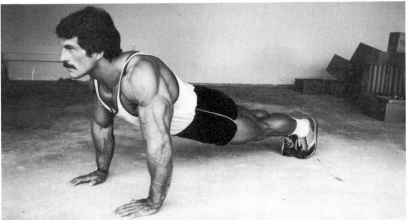

Exercise No. 3—Push-ups

Muscles Exercised—Chest

Comment—I find push-ups very rewarding psychologically and they produce great results very quickly. And they are especially good for women because they firm and tone the entire pectoral area without increasing bust size.

Directions—Lie on the floor face down and place your hands on the floor beside your shoulders. Your toes should be tucked in. Now push yourself off the floor by straightening your arms. Keep your back and legs straight. When your arms are fully extended your body should be in a straight line. Hold the arms-extended position for the count of two and then slowly lower yourself until your chest—and only your chest—touches the floor. Repeat twelve times.

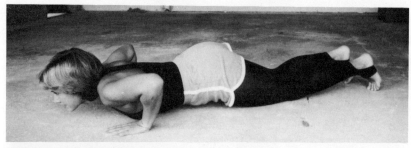

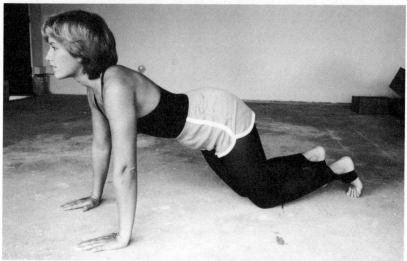

If you find the regular push-up too difficult at first, try this less strenuous half push-up. Take the same starting position described for the regular push-up but when you push up with your arms, keep your knees and lower legs on the floor. This way you're raising only your torso and it's much easier. After a few workouts you'll be ready for the real thing.

Reminder—When doing either style push-up keep your back straight throughout and don't let your upper body rest in the lowered position.

Exercise No. 4—Press Behind Neck

MUSCLES EXERCISED—Shoulders

Comment—This is one of the most widely practiced and productive of all shoulder exercises and another favorite of mine. It

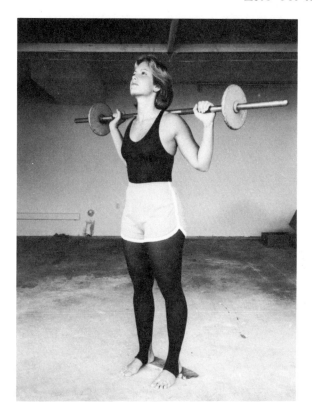

works the entire deltoid area (the thick muscle covering the shoulder joint), the trapezius (on the top of the shoulders), the upper back, and the triceps (behind the biceps), so it's really a multiple-muscle exercise.

Directions—Begin with your feet about shoulder-width apart, making sure you have a firm base. Bend over and grasp the barbell with an overhand, shoulder-width grip. Then raise it over your head and lower it so it rests on your shoulders. Your elbows should be pointing directly out to the side. From the shoulders, "press" the weight slowly and deliberately over your head, pause at the top, and slowly lower. Repeat twelve times.

Reminder—Be sure to keep the back straight and the head up. Look at that point where the wall and ceiling meet.

Hint—Use light weights until you get the form down pat. Too much weight can cause you to lose control of the bar.

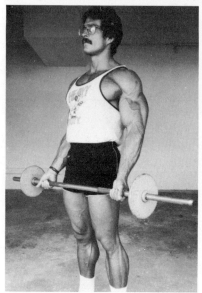

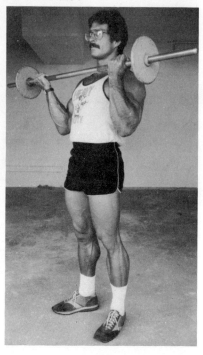

Exercise No. 5—Curls

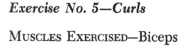

MUSCLES EXERCISED—Biceps

Comment—The barbell curl is probably the simplest of the bicep exercises but it produces quick results. It may be the old Charles Atlas syndrome but people tend to judge muscular development by the size of the bicep.

Directions—With your feet spread about shoulder-width, bend over, grasp the barbell with an underhand (palms up) grip. Place your hands about shoulder-width apart. Now stand up holding the bar with the arms extended, elbows at the sides, and the back straight. "Curl" the bar to the top of your chest keeping the elbows close to your sides where they can act as pivots. Pause at the top and then slowly lower the weight, keeping it under control at all times. Repeat twelve times.

Reminder—It's easy to slip into a loose style while doing curls so pay careful attention to form and try to execute all the repetitions properly. Keep the shoulders straight. Don't lean back for that extra leverage. Don't let the bar fall back to the starting position.

Hint—Keep body movement at a minimum. This will prevent any upper or lower back strain.

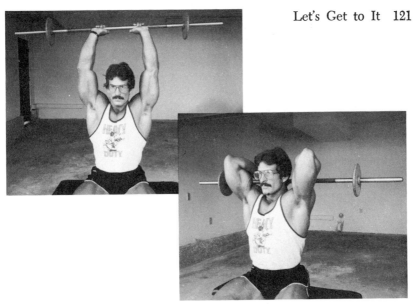

Exercise No. 6—Tricep Extension

MUSCLES EXERCISED—Triceps

Comment—This exercise has a very direct effect on the tricep, the muscle on the back of your upper arm, directly behind the bicep. Strength in the upper arms is very good for most sports activities and the triceps play an important role in such movements as throwing and swimming strokes.

Directions—Place your feet about shoulder-width apart (or sit on a bench), bend and grasp the barbell in an overhand grip with your hands six to ten inches apart. Bring the bar to a position directly over your head. From there, slowly lower it behind your head, keeping your elbows tucked in near your ears and acting as pivots. Lower the weight as far as you can toward the back of your neck. Raise back to the starting position. Repeat twelve times.

Reminder—Keep your back straight and head up as usual. Keep the elbows in or you'll find yourself doing another set of behind the neck presses.

Hint—Watch the amount of weight you use for this exercise. It's much more difficult than the shoulder press. Better underestimate your strength on this one.

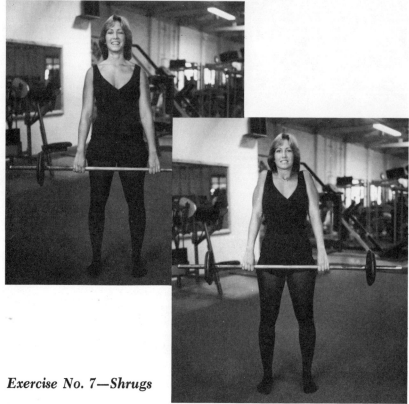

Exercise No. 7—Shrugs

MUSCLES EXERCISED—Trapezius

Comment—The trapezius is a beautifully designed sheath of muscle that spans the upper back and is attached to the base of the skull, making it possible to raise the head and shoulders. Tension build-up in this area often results in stiff necks and tension headaches. Shrugs work the trapezius and help to relieve tension build-up.

Directions—Stand facing the bar with your feet comfortably spread, ankles actually touching the bar. Reach down and grasp the bar with an overhand, shoulder-width grip. Stand up, letting the bar hang at arm's length. Shrug your shoulders straight up and try to touch your ears with the tops of your shoulders. Hold the shrug position for a count of two and then lower your shoulders back to their normal position. Repeat twelve times.

Reminder—Try to keep your shoulders back and your chest out.

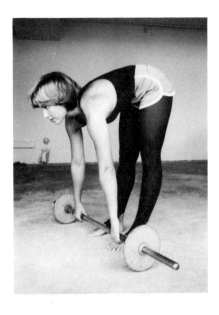

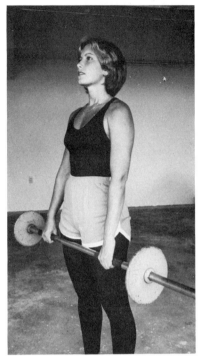

Exercise No. 8—Dead Lifts

MUSCLES EXERCISED—Lower Back

Comment—Lower back problems rank as one of the most common medical complaints, especially in athletes. In fact, almost everyone experiences some form of back pain at one time or another. And there are few problems that hinder physical activity more than backache. Dead lifts provide the best form of exercise for the lower back, strengthening the muscles in the area and relieving tension.

Directions—Take the same starting position as you did for the shrugs. Bend forward at the waist, bending the knees just slightly, and grasp the bar with an overhand grip, hands shoulder-width apart. With head up, stand erect with the bar, keeping the arms straight and the shoulders back. Now, keeping your knees as straight as possible, bend over and lower the weight slowly until it touches the floor. Repeat twelve times.

Hint—Use light weights and pay careful attention to proper execution of the dead lifts, especially if you have been inactive for some time. For the greatest benefit be sure to exaggerate the shoulder movement when you reach the standing position.

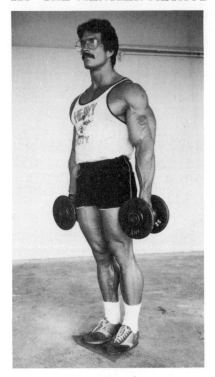

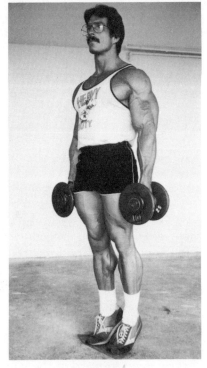

Exercise No. 9—Toe Raises

MUSCLES EXERCISED—Calves

Comment—The simple toe raise is still the best exercise for strengthening the calf muscles. These muscles are disproportionately strong for their size and can take a lot of exercise.

Direction—Stand straight with your hands on your hips and your feet a few inches apart. Keeping your body in a straight line, raise up on your toes as far as you possibly can, hold for a count of two, and lower your heels back to the floor. (You may want to hold light dumbbells at your sides for this exercise.) Repeat twelve times.

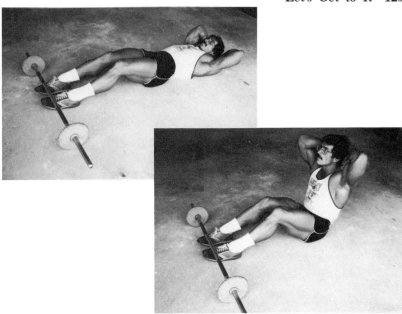

Exercise No. 10—Sit-ups

Muscles Exercised—Stomach

Comment—This is the old standby. It's the one we've all done at one time or another but it's still a highly effective stomach tightener.

Directions—Lie flat on your back on a mat or a pillow. Flex your knees until you can put your feet flat on the floor. Tuck your toes under a couch, bed, or barbell. Clasp your hands behind your head and curl your body up from the waist until your elbows touch your raised knees. Then slowly uncurl and lower yourself back to the mat. Start with ten repetitions and try to add one a day. When you can virtually do as many sit-ups as you want without undue strain, you can increase the intensity of the exercise by holding a light weight behind your neck.

Reminder—Use your stomach muscles as much as possible. The strain should be in your stomach, not in your legs or back.

Hint—Pause for the count of one at the completion of each sit-up to prevent bouncing. The muscles, especially the lower abdominal muscles, should be doing the work, not momentum.

Cool-downs—Approximately Fifteen Minutes

Most of the warm-up exercises are also good for your cool-down period but especially the arm circles, toe touches, bends, and twists. Do them all at moderate speed, consciously slowing your movements after about five minutes. Walking is a very effective method of slowing your body down and dissipating the energy build-up you've established. Do *not* jump into a hot or cold shower immediately after completing your workout. Stay on your feet even if it's only to look out the window. To repeat: Don't stop and flop.

As I said before, I think it's advisable to continue this break-in routine for at least one week even if you're in great physical shape. If you're in less than top condition, two to four weeks will be better. This is something you'll have to judge for yourself. Just don't try to go too far too fast. This isn't a race. You're only competing with yourself and you will be the winner if you take your time.

Chapter 4

Stepping Up

By now I'm sure you're already seeing some changes in your body, some new firmness here and a little more shape there. You've probably dropped a couple of pounds, maybe even tightened up your belt a notch. And I know you feel better mentally as well. You've started to take some action, to battle the bulges and you're even telling your friends about this great new thing you're doing. And a lot of the nervous tension is gone too, simply drained away as you physically exert yourself. It's a great feeling.

Now that you're ready, let's take a step up the ladder and add some intensity and a few new exercises to your routine.

The format will stay the same—warm-up, intense exercises, cool-down. As before, you'll be exercising the larger muscles at the beginning of each session when you have more energy available. But from now on each workout should begin with a pulse reading. A second reading should be taken after your warm-up and a third after you've completed the first two exercises. Take your pulse again after the fourth exercise, after the sixth, and so on, and then one final time after the cool-down period. This is quite a lot of pulse taking, I know, but in a short time you'll be able to sense your heart rate and at that point you'll only need to document it at the beginning, in the middle, and at the end of each session. If at any time you feel your pulse getting out of control, exceeding the maximum rate you've set, it's best to reevaluate that rate and very possibly lower it. The pulse taking is a good safety valve, so take it as often as you need to.

Be sure you don't rest more than thirty seconds between sets of exercises and that the weights you've selected are not too light. You won't be able to sustain the cardiovascular training effect if the large muscle groups are not taxed.

Charting Your Progress

If you diligently follow the suggested workouts in this chapter and the Mentzer 3,500 Weight-Control Program, your progress should be almost immediate. As I said, I'm sure you noticed progress even during the break-in period. If, however, your progress isn't steady (allowing for a plateau here and there) you may be doing something wrong. The most common mistakes are:

1) Resting too long between sets
2) Using weights that are too heavy or too light
3) Poor form
4) Skipping workouts

Any of these mistakes can slow up progress, *especially skipping workouts*. A combination of them can negate progress entirely.

The Mentzer Method Progress Chart (see page 130) will help take the guesswork out of your record keeping. By using the chart you'll be able to keep a continuous record including the date of your workout, the amount of weight used for each exercise, the number of repetitions for each, and your pulse rate. Analyze your progress periodically (not every day because changes don't show that quickly) to make sure your weights are increasing and your pulse rate is decreasing. What's actually happening is that the training is increasing cardiac output and strengthening the entire cardiovascular system. This will eventually allow your heart to work more economically even under the stress of exercise. This means a slower heart rate, a lower oxygen demand, and a decreased energy drain.

To achieve this new level of fitness you have to be committed to progress. You can't dog it. If you're not willing to expend the required energy, you'll be doing nothing but setting up a pattern of failure, frustration, and a certain amount of anxiety. If you are committed, you will succeed. I can say this unequivocally because "success" is measured by your own personal standard. You may not be lifting as much as the next person, but your heart rate will slow, you'll lose weight and you'll feel better.

Exercise Sequences

As the amount of weight you use increases and the rest time you take between exercises decreases, you'll be firmly on the road to a high level of physical fitness. At this point one sequence of intense exercises will take only about ten minutes, less than the required twelve to fifteen minutes of stimulation the heart needs for a cardiovascular training benefit. A second sequence will have to be added to increase the work load. This will effectively maintain your high pulse rate and further stimulate skeletal-muscle development. As the body continues to adapt to the intensity of the work load—becoming stronger and more fit with a lower pulse rate—you will have to repeat the first two sequences or, if you're working out in a gym, add the suggested third sequence. The first two groups of exercises can be performed by anyone with a minimum of conventional weight-training equipment. The third sequence requires specialized equipment. I'm including the third group for those people who are working out in a well-equipped gym or a Nautilus facility and for those who now might want to consider gym or Nautilus workouts.

The intense-exercise sequences suggested here can be added progressively over time as your level of fitness continues to increase. I'd say at least one month (that's only twelve workouts) should be spent on the first sequence before even considering the second. But everyone's progress will be different, so make your own judgments. Just don't be afraid to go forward—or back, for that matter—as your body dictates.

First Sequence

Most of the exercises in this sequence will be familiar from the break-in period so refer to the previous chapter if you need

Progress Chart

STARTING DATE ————

WEIGHT ————

MEASUREMENTS

Chest ————
Biceps ————
Waist ————
Hips ————
Thighs ————

DATE	EXERCISES			PULSE					
	Sequence	Weight	Reps	Resting	After Warmup	After 2 Exer.	After 4 Exer.	After 6 Exer.	After Cool-Down

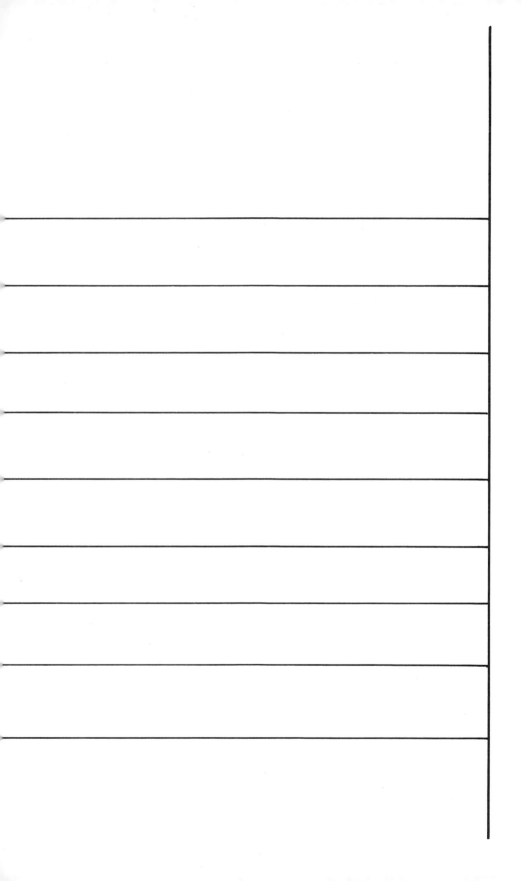

to refresh your memory on any point. You can continue to use the warm-up and cool-down exercises suggested in Chapter 3, adding any of the variations you've developed on your own. Here is the order of the first sequence:

1) Lunges; 2) Toe Raises; 3) Barbell Rows; 4) Dead Lifts; 5) Bench Presses; 6) Press Behind Neck; 7) Curls; 8) Tricep Extensions; 9) Sit-ups. Do ten to twelve repetitions of each exercise.

The new exercises in this First Sequence and exercises that vary in any appreciable way from the previous chapter are described below.

Exercise No. 1—Lunges

Muscles Exercised—Thighs

Comment—This is an extremely good exercise for the entire thigh, both the quadricep in front and the hamstring in back. I think it's best to use only the bar for this exercise in the beginning, adding weight when you're completely comfortable with the movements involved.

Directions—Stand erect with your feet a few inches apart. Bend over and grip the bar overhand with the hands slightly more than shoulder-width apart. Press the bar over your head, slowly lower it behind your neck, and rest it on your shoulders. Adjust

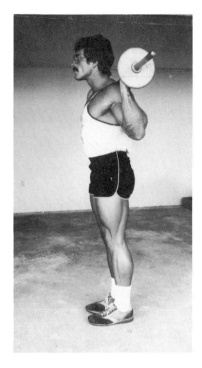

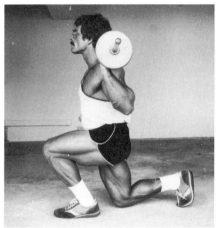

the bar so that it's well balanced and comfortable. Now "thrust" by stepping forward with your left foot about two and one-half feet, planting it firmly flat on the floor. Keep your back straight but let your right heel come off the floor as you bring your right knee as close to the floor as possible, touching it if you can. You'll feel the thigh muscles in both legs stretching. Hold that position—back straight, left foot flat, right knee touching the floor, right heel raised—for a count of two. Push back to the starting position and thrust forward with the left foot bringing the right knee to the floor. Do ten to twelve thrusts for each leg.

Reminder—Balance is important and may be difficult at first so experiment without the bar if necessary until you find the forward stride that's best for you. As you gain strength and flexibility you'll increase your stride and need heavier weights.

Hint—You'll be able to keep your back straight if you keep your eyes on that point where the ceiling meets the wall.

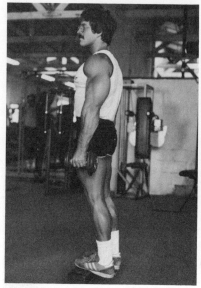

Exercise No. 2—Toe Raises

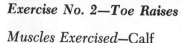

*Muscles Exercised—*Calf

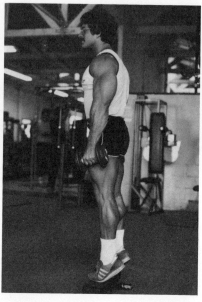

*Directions—*The toe raises are essentially the same as those described in the Break-in chapter except now you'll be adding more weight and using a block of wood under your toes. Stand with your arms at your sides with a fairly heavy dumbbell in each hand. Step up onto the wood block (a short piece of two-by-four will do the job) and balance on your toes, letting your heels touch the floor if possible. Keep your body in a straight line and lock your knees. Now raise up on your toes as high as you can, hold at the top for a count of two, and slowly lower your heels back to the floor.

*Reminder—*Balance may be a problem here, too, so practice without weights if necessary until you get the hang of it.

*Hint—*The calves are very strong so don't hesitate to add weight quickly.

Exercise No. 3—Barbell Rows
*Directions—*See Break-in Chapter.

Exercise No. 4—Dead Lifts
*Directions—*See Break-in Chapter.

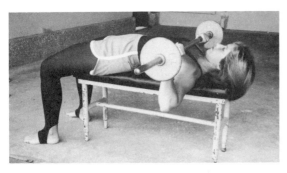

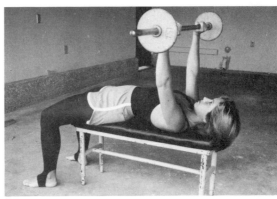

Exercise No. 5—Bench Presses

Muscles Exercised—Pectorals and Triceps

Comment—This is a fine exercise for the entire upper body. The pectorals, triceps, and shoulder muscles (deltoids) are all brought into play so eventually you'll probably be able to handle quite a bit of weight. At first it's best to practice with a relatively light weight because, though the press seems simple, it takes a certain amount of skill to raise and lower the weight, keeping it under control at all times.

Directions—Grasp the bar with an overhand grip, hands about shoulder-width apart. Press it to your chest and slowly sit down on the end of the bench. Lower yourself until your back is flat on the bench and your head is resting comfortably. Your feet should be flat on the floor for leverage. From this position press the weight straight up, pause at the top, and lower it, keeping it under control until the bar touches your chest. Your elbows will be below the line of the bench.

Reminder—Your buttocks should remain on the bench at all times during this exercise and there should be a slight arch in your back.

Hint—When you begin to use heavier weights, bench presses are much easier if you have a partner hand you the bar after you've taken the arms-extended position on the bench. If you have a bench with brackets to support the bar, you won't have to worry about this problem. If you don't have a bench at all, you can use the floor but the benefits won't be as great because you won't be able to lower the bar all the way to your chest.

Exercise No. 6—Press Behind Neck

Directions—See Break-in Chapter.

Exercise No. 7—Tricep Extensions

Directions—See Break-in Chapter.

Exercise No. 8—Sit-ups

Directions—See Break-in Chapter.

Second Sequence

Order of exercises: 1) Squats; 2) Toe Raises; 3) Shrugs; 4) Upright Rows; 5) Alternate Dumbbell Presses; 6) Dumbbell Flys; 7) Alternate Dumbbell Curls; 8) Lying Tricep Extensions; 9) Leg Raises. Do ten to twelve repetitions of each exercise.

Exercise No. 1—Squats

Directions—See Break-in Chapter.

Exercise No. 2—Toe Raises

Directions—See First Sequence.

Exercise No. 3—Shrugs

Directions—See Break-in Chapter.

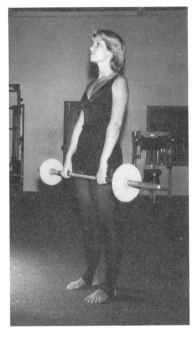
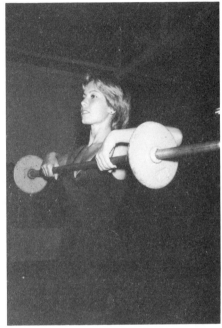

Exercise No. 4—Upright Rows

Muscles Exercised—Trapezius, Deltoids, and Biceps.

Comment—Upright rows are an economical exercise because three muscles are worked at the same time, and the entire upper body reaps the benefits. After you complete the shrugs, move directly into the upright rows, using the same stance and grip as you did for the shrugs. From the arm-extended position, lift the bar along the plane of the body until it's just under your chin. Pause for a count of two and lower it slowly to the starting position.

Reminder—Try not to jerk or swing the bar. Keep it smooth.

Hint—In the top position your elbows should be as high as your ears. If you can't get that high, you're using too much weight.

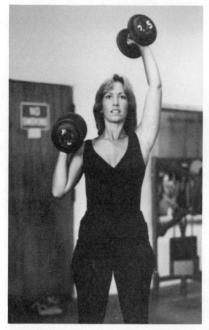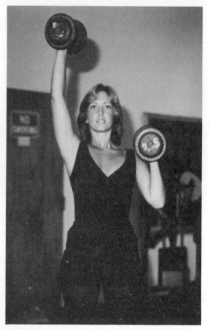

Exercise No. 5—Alternate Dumbbell Presses

Muscles Exercised—Shoulders

Comment—This exercise benefits the same muscles as the press behind the neck but it gives variety in working the shoulder area and it's good for flexibility.

Directions—Stand straight with your feet comfortably spread. Bend over, pick up one dumbbell in each hand, and raise them to your shoulders. Your elbows should be pointed straight out from your sides. Now "press" the dumbbell by raising your right arm straight up until it's fully extended. Keep the left arm in the lowered position. When you reach the top with the right arm it should be close to your head. Now lower it slowly and at the same time begin to press the left arm. Continue to alternate arms until you've completed ten repetitions with each arm.

Reminder—Keep your back straight, your head up, and your shoulders well back.

Hint—Use a moderately heavy weight because you can handle it.

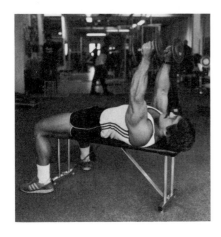

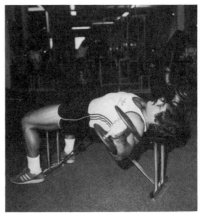

Exercise No. 6—Dumbbell Flys

Muscles Exercised—Pectorals

Comment—This is an especially good exercise for women because it helps to keep the bustline high and firm. For men it gives the pectorals a more defined look.

Directions—Grasp a dumbbell in each hand as you did for the alternate dumbbell presses and then lie down on the bench with your feet firmly on the floor, your back straight, and your head comfortable. Bring the dumbbells together (your knuckles should be facing) over your upper chest. Keep your arms almost fully extended but maintain an angle at the elbow. This will keep the stress on the pectorals instead of transferring part of it to the triceps and it takes the strain off the elbows. Lower the dumbbells slowly outward until your arms are parallel with the floor. Lower the weights a little farther toward the floor if you can. Raise them back to the starting position. Try to keep the angle of the elbows constant throughout the exercise.

Reminder—Don't let the dumbbells just fall to the side. Keep them under control, and parallel to each other all the time.

Hint—This exercise can be done on the floor.

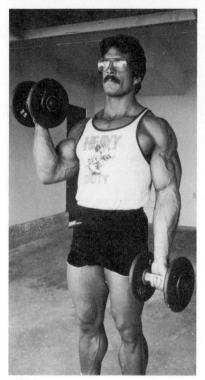 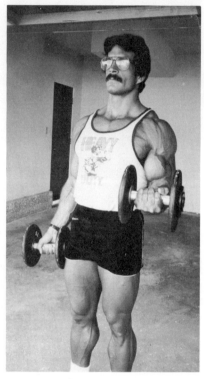

Exercise No. 7—Alternate Dumbbell Curls

Muscles Exercised—Biceps

Comment—I like this exercise because it adds variety to the workout.

Directions—Bend over and grasp one dumbbell in each hand. Stand straight up, arms extended at your sides, palms facing forward. Keeping your left arm down, "curl" your right arm to your right shoulder. As you slowly lower the right arm to the starting position, begin to raise the left. Keep alternating until you've completed ten repetitions with each arm.

Reminder—Keep your back straight and try not to yank the dumbbells up from the bottom.

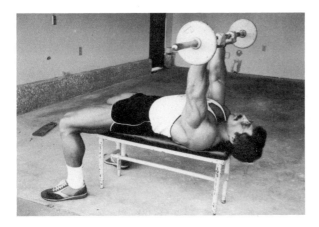

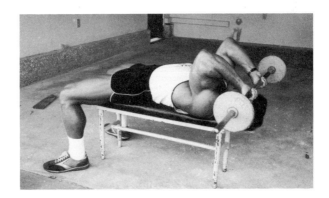

Exercise No. 8—Lying Tricep Extensions

Muscles Exercised—Triceps

Directions—Bend over and grasp the bar with an overhand grip, hands about twelve inches apart. Lift the bar to your chest and then slowly take the standard position on the bench. Press the weight to the arms-extended position, then slowly lower it toward your head while bending your elbows. Continue to lower the bar until your elbows are pointing at the ceiling. Return to the starting position and repeat six times.

Reminder—Keep your elbows as close together as you can.

Hint—As you lower the weight let your back arch off the bench but at the same time try to keep your buttocks from lifting.

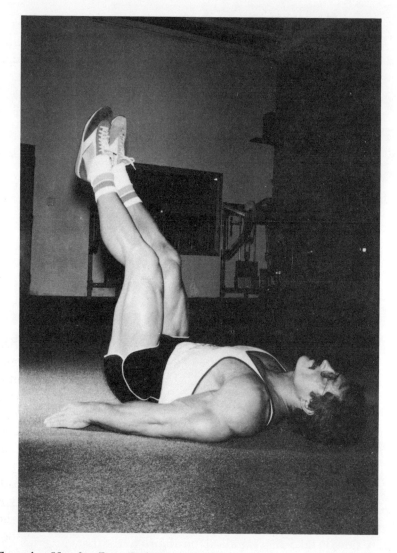

Exercise No. 9—Leg Raises

*Muscles Exercised—*Stomach

*Comment—*Like sit-ups, this exercise is an old standby but it is nevertheless an effective tummy tightener that works especially well on the area around the navel where poor muscle tone causes the most unsightly bulges, rolls, and wrinkles.

Directions—Lie flat on your back on an exercise mat or with a pillow under your buttocks. Put your arms at your sides, palms pressed on the floor for stability. Keeping your legs as straight as possible, knees and feet together, slowly raise both legs at the same time until they are as nearly perpendicular to the floor as you can get them. Then lower them slowly back to the floor. Repeat ten times and try to add one a day.

Reminder—Keep your legs as straight as possible; lock the knees if you can.

Hint—Don't let your heels quite touch the floor when lowering the legs. This provides just a little more intensity.

Third Sequence

This sequence of exercises, as I said, requires some specialized equipment. Any fully equipped gym will have what you need. If you don't want to head for the gym or the Nautilus center, just do those exercises you can (you're already familiar with them by now) with the equipment you have at home. Be sure to do them in the order as shown because, as before, they work the large muscles first when you have the most energy. Keep in mind that this third sequence radically boosts the intensity of your workout, so don't tackle them until you're absolutely ready. Believe me, it's better to repeat the first two sequences in your workouts two and even three times before moving up. But when you're ready, give it a try. The three sequences should take about forty minutes the first few times through, but you will be able to work yourself down to thirty minutes in a relatively short time.

Order of exercises: 1) Leg Extensions; 2) Squats; 3) Leg Curls; 4) Leg Press; 5) Bent-arm Pullovers; 6) Lat Pull-down; 7) Barbell Rows; 8) Shrugs; 9) Upright Rows; 10) Dumbbell Lateral Raise; 11) Curls; 13) Tricep Extensions.

The new exercises in this sequence are described on the following pages.

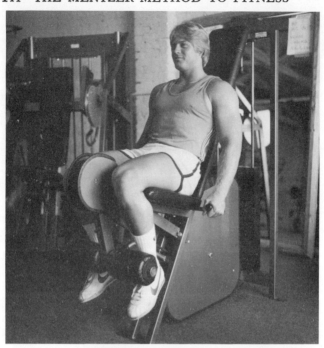

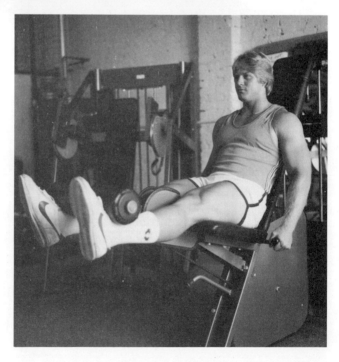

Exercise No. 1—Leg Extensions

Muscles Exercised—Thighs

Comment—This exercise provides the most direct stress for the frontal thigh muscles, the quadriceps. Unlike squats, which work the entire thigh, these extensions isolate the frontal thigh area and promote rapid development.

Directions—Sit on the seat of the leg-extension machine keeping your buttocks and thighs against it at all times. Place your ankles under the pads. Grip the handles but don't try to crush them. Now raise your legs slowly and smoothly until they are parallel with the floor. Pause and lower slowly. Repeat six times.

Reminder—Because of the relative delicacy of the knees, this exercise must be performed carefully and in good form.

Hint—Lock the knees when your legs are parallel with the floor. This will give you complete control during the negative movement. Don't press on the handles; they're only for stability.

Exercise No. 2—Squats

Directions—See Break-in Chapter

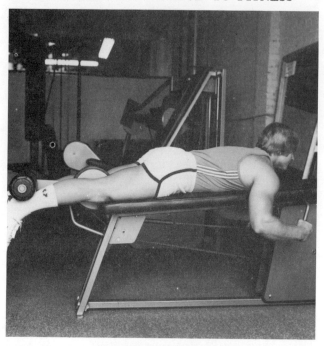

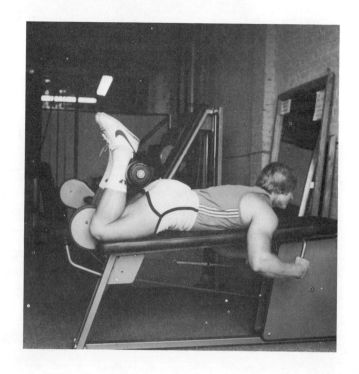

Exercise No. 3—Leg Curls

Muscles Exercised—Hamstrings

Comment—Leg curls work the hamstring muscles on the back of the legs behind the thighs. It's important that you develop strength in these leg biceps to counterbalance the power of the frontal thighs. Hamstrings are highly susceptible to pulls and tears if the quadriceps on the front of the thighs are allowed to become proportionately stronger. Most of the leg exercises you've been doing are good for the thighs but the leg curls directly stimulate the hamstrings and shouldn't be neglected. This exercise is also good for firming the buttocks.

Directions—Lie perfectly flat on the bench, face down, with your knees just over the edge. Put your feet under the roller pads and hold the handles lightly to keep the body steady. Curl your legs up as far as you can and try to touch the heels to the buttocks. When your legs are in the top position, pause for a count of two, and slowly lower them back to the starting position. Repeat six times.

Reminder—If you can't curl close to the buttocks, you are probably using too much weight, and if you can't hold the weight at the top, you didn't raise it through muscular contraction alone. Try not to use momentum to carry the weight.

Hint—Flex the top of the foot toward the knee throughout the exercise.

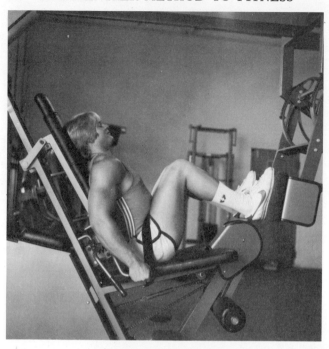

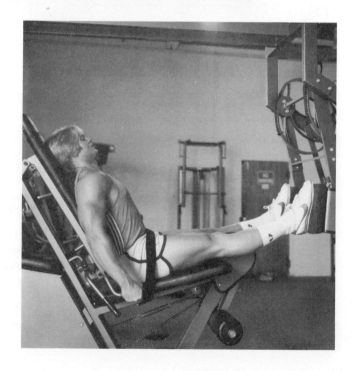

Exercise No. 4—Leg Press

Muscles Exercised—All Thigh Muscles, Hamstrings, and Buttocks

Comment—Leg presses are especially good for stimulating muscle growth because of the natural power of the legs and the heavy weights you can use in this movement. At one time I was having some trouble developing mass on the outer sweep of my thighs and turned to leg presses for the answer. I eventually got to the point where I could do eight repetitions using 1,100 pounds and my thigh problems were over.

Directions—Sit on the seat of the leg extension machine and belt yourself in. Hold the handles for leverage and balance, and, bending your knees, place your feet about twelve inches apart on the footpad. Press forward until your knees are straight and your legs fully extended. Slowly bring the weight back to the starting position. Repeat six times.

Reminder—As with leg extensions, proper form is important because of the delicacy of the knees. Don't lock your knees in the extended position.

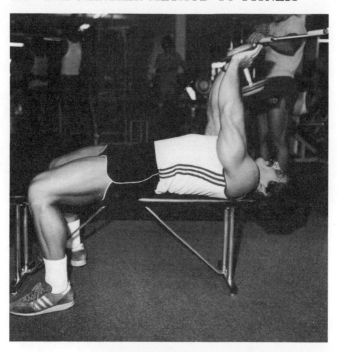

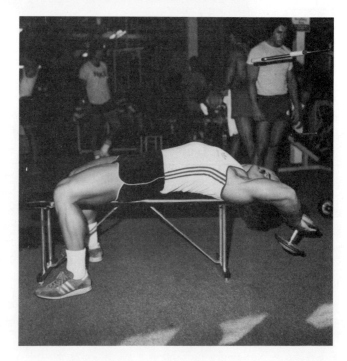

Exercise No. 5—Bent-arm Pullovers

Muscles Exercised—Latissimus Dorsi

Comment—This exercise works the thorax and the breathing muscles in the chest as well as the lats and it even benefits the stomach muscles. It's a multiple conditioner.

Directions—Lie flat on the bench with your head and neck over the edge, feet flat on the floor. Hold a light dumbbell directly over your head with both hands. Take a deep breath and lower the weight behind your head to a point slightly below the level of the bench. Keep your elbows bent outward at about a 45-degree angle throughout the movement to reduce strain. Return to the starting position and repeat six times.

Reminder—Lower the weight as far as you can but stop when you feel a stretch in your shoulders.

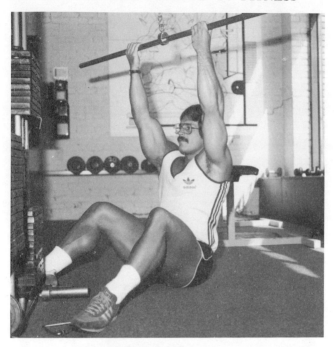

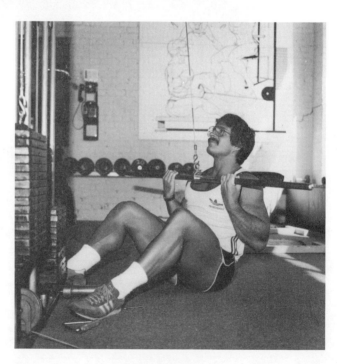

Exercise No. 6—Lat Pull-down

Muscles Exercised—Latissimus Dorsi and Biceps

Comment—This is a very effective exercise for the lats and though it works the biceps indirectly, it still provides a positive benefit for them.

Directions—Sit directly under the bar with your feet comfortably spread on the floor. Reach up and grasp the bar in an underhand, shoulder-width grip. Pull the bar straight down in a plane with your chest until it is around the mid-chest level. Hold it there for a count of two and then slowly return the weight to the starting position. Repeat six times.

Reminder—Remain seated at all times during this exercise. If you have to raise up, you're probably using too much weight. Select a weight that allows you to pull the bar as far as your chest.

Hint—If you don't have access to a professional lat pull-down machine, you can substitute an extra set of pullovers.

Exercise No. 7—Barbell Rows

Directions—See Break-in Chapter

Exercise No. 8—Shrugs

Directions—See Break-in Chapter

Exercise No. 9—Upright Rows

Directions—See Second Sequence

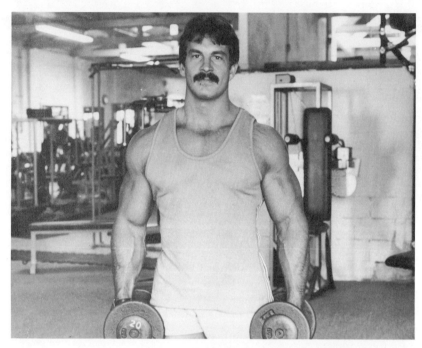

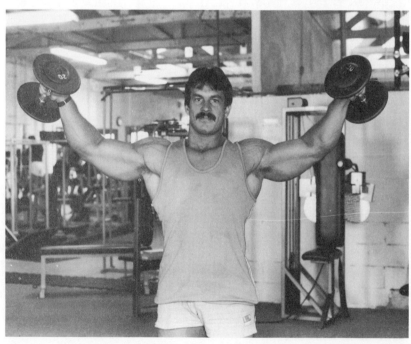

Exercise No. 10—Dumbbell Lateral Raise

Muscles Exercised—Shoulders

Comment—No exercise beats this one for strengthening and widening the shoulders. Even if you have narrow clavicles these lateral movements will markedly increase the size of your shoulders.

Directions—With your feet comfortably apart, bend over and pick up a dumbbell in each hand. Then stand straight with the dumbbells at your sides in the arms-extended position, palms facing thighs. Keeping your head and back straight, slowly raise your arms out to the sides with arms and elbows as straight as possible. When your arms are parallel with the floor, pause for a count of two and slowly lower them back to the starting position. Repeat six times.

Reminder—Don't raise up on your toes or swing the dumbbells up. Use your shoulder muscles.

Hint—Start with fairly light weights.

Exercise No. 11—Curls

Directions—See Break-in Chapter

Exercise No. 12—Tricep Extensions

Direction—See Break-in Chapter

A Final Word

I'm sure you've noticed that I haven't suggested any time limits on these exercise sequences. I did this purposely because I have no way of knowing how fast you'll progress and neither do you. That's why I haven't said follow Sequence One for six weeks, Sequence Two for four weeks, and so on. It doesn't make any sense. Everyone's body is different. Muscles respond differently to the stimulus of resistance exercises. Fatigue and soreness can be factors in your development. The intensity of these exercises is something you'll have to get used to. This, after all, isn't just any exercise program. So I won't say that in six weeks you'll be bending steel bars with your bare hands. But I will guarantee you that in a very short time you'll be able to see and feel the difference. Your body will begin to take a new shape and your general state of health and well-being will be enhanced markedly. How fast this happens is up to you. But above all, be patient and realistic. Stick with it and you'll soon see what the Mentzer Method of weight training and weight control can do for you. Before very, long this program will become part of your lifestyle.

Good luck. I know you can do it.

Chapter 5

The Serious Bodybuilder

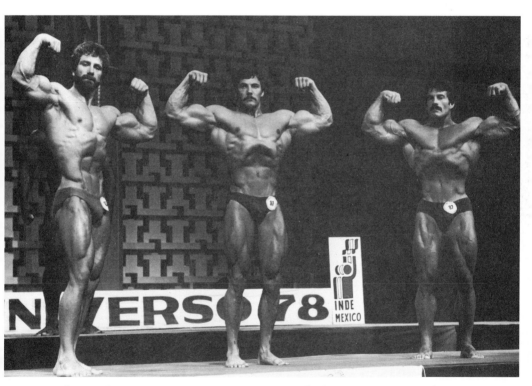

The 1978 Mr. Universe contest in Acapulco, Mexico. From left to right: *Josef Wilcocz, Germany, second place; Reid Schindle, Canada, third place; and Mike Mentzer, United States, Mr. Universe, with a perfect score of 300 points.*

Since winning the 1976 Mr. America contest in the Felt Forum at Madison Square Garden, I've had the opportunity to talk with thousands of bodybuilders about their goals and aspirations. These people are not just interested in improving their appearance, they're serious about developing outstanding physiques, entering contests, winning titles. These conversations have given me a much better understanding of why people fail in bodybuilding programs. I can sum it up in two words: unrealistic expectations.

Realism

Common sense will tell you that to build muscle tissue beyond normal levels is a slow process that requires dedication and work. Yet it's not unusual to find bodybuilders who actually expect to gain a pound of muscle a day. It obviously can't be done and it's this lack of realism that leads to disappointment and frustration, and ultimately to failure. If, in fact, it was possible to gain even a pound of muscle tissue a week, a little basic math shows that you would pick up more than fifty pounds of muscle a year. It's ludicrous, I know, but I'm amazed at how many people expect that kind of progress. Actually, a ten-pound muscle gain in a year is a considerable achievement. It may not sound like much to a would-be Mr. America, but at that rate you could gain fifty pounds of muscle in five years or enough to transform a 160-pounder into a title contender of 210 pounds—my weight when I won the Mr. Universe title.

Danny Padilla is a good case in point. He weighed a very impressive 165 when he won the lightweight Mr. Universe title in 1978. He told me that when he started bodybuilding more than ten years ago he weighed 120 and was so slight that he had given serious thought to losing a few pounds and becoming a jockey. His gain of forty-five pounds over a ten-year training career represents an average yearly gain of only 4½ pounds, or about six ounces, less than half a pound, a month. This should offer some hope to those disappointed with similar gains because Danny is now one of the most muscular men I've ever met.

Put bluntly, it's only this kind of long-range commitment—ten years or more—that results in any worthwhile alteration of your appearance. No one has yet built a Mr. Universe physique overnight. Great athletes in all sports must train hard for years. Bodybuilding is no exception.

Genetics

Bodybuilders tend to be among the most fanatical of athletes. They are willing to spend endless hours in the gym, eat any combination of strange-sounding, and even stranger-tasting food, and pop pills in their quest to develop title-winning physiques. I've seen some give up family, career, and education to pursue their bodybuilding goals.

What makes this effort so tragic is that for most people this is another unrealistic goal. They simply don't have the genetic makeup, the raw physical potential, to become Mr. America or a Mr. Anything. What most bodybuilders fail to realize is that the title winners, the people they look to for guidance in the science of bodybuilding, were genetically predisposed to develop large, shapely muscles and that their achievements are often made in spite of their training methods. There have been a number of studies which show that an athlete's strength, speed, and endurance are a matter of genetic endowment and no amount of training can overcome this deficiency in the genes.

Look at Arnold Schwarzenegger. His training and dietary practices are among the most widely publicized in bodybuilding. If it was just his training and diet that were responsible for his great success, there should be an entire army of Schwarzeneggers since most bodybuilders train as he does. His principles have been followed by thousands of bodybuilders for more than ten years now and there is still only one Arnold. Why? Genetics.

Per-Olof Astrand, the Swedish expert in work and exercise physiology, says, "A person's potential for development of muscle strength is determined at birth . . . and remains unaltered throughout life. It may not be quite fair, but it is nevertheless a fact that the 'choice of parents' is important for athletic achievement."

The O. J. Simpsons, Hank Aarons, Marty Liquoris, Nadia Comanecis, and Arnold Schwarzeneggers all inherited certain traits that enabled them to excel and eventually dominate their sports. But ability and physical capacity alone aren't of much use unless the individual is motivated and willing to use all of his or her endowment to the limit. In other words, you have to work at it. This combination of special gifts and motivation is rare, and this is what makes the super athlete such a wonder.

I realize that no serious bodybuilder is going to stop dreaming no matter what I say, and I guess that's good because regardless of hereditary limitations, significant progress can be made by anyone. And since there isn't a thing we can do about those genetic limitations, there is no point in worrying about them.

Assess Your Potential

While potential refers to possibility and can be finally determined only in retrospect, there are a number of tangible physical traits that offer a fairly accurate suggestion of what a person's physical potential may be.

The most visible of these physical characteristics is the skeletal structure. The size and strength of the skeleton determine the actual amount of muscle a person can ultimately support as well as certain aesthetic qualities. For example, the relative size of the clavicles and the pelvis will determine whether the development of the classic V-taper is possible.

Muscle length determines the ultimate size of muscle development. The longer the muscle the greater its potential for acquiring mass. The length of the bone to which the muscle is attached is of no real importance. Taller people, of course, have longer bones and therefore longer muscles but their muscles have no greater ability for developing mass. Even within one individual (let alone a species) there is variation. For example, a person with full-length biceps doesn't necessarily possess full-length calves. Lou Ferrigno, a two-time winner of the Mr. Universe title and a television star as the Incredible Hulk, has long upper-arm muscles which take great mass, but his calves are very high on his lower leg and this limits their mass potential. It's extremely rare to find a person with great potential for muscle development over the entire body. Sergio Oliva, a bodybuilder with even greater potential than Arnold, is the only person I can recall who was able to develop extraordinary muscular mass proportionately in all body parts.

A less tangible trait that needs to be assessed if you want to know your potential for muscular development is the density of muscle, the number of muscle fibers. Here again, heredity is the governing factor. The number of muscle fibers is determined before birth. This number is unchangeable. You cannot add muscle fiber.

Body type is also a factor in overall physical development. The ectomorph is slight, reedlike from the side, with long, thin hands and fingers, a tendency to develop long, stringy muscles, and with low fat-storage capacity, the type of person who will always be thin even without dieting. The mesomorph is the football type with broad shoulders, a deep chest, heavy bones, sturdy legs, well-formed muscles, and a medium capacity for fat storage. The endomorph is almost the opposite of the ectomorph, with softly rounded body, narrow sloping shoulders, pudgy hands and feet, and high capacity for fat storage—the typical pear shape.

Very few people are exclusively one of the three body types, though certainly one type tends to dominate. If you're a bodybuilder and think you're an ectomorph, don't despair. Arnold was a tall, gangly ectomorphic type before he took up bodybuilding. But you have to be realistic. If you have a physique like Woody Allen's, you're not likely to become a linebacker for the Chicago Bears or a Mr. Universe.

Let's take stock. It's clear you can't change your body type, your skeleton, the amount of muscle fiber, or the length of your muscles. These realities will place certain limits on your potential. What then is possible?

Fortunately, your ultimate potential can't be assessed now and you'll never know what you might have achieved unless you train hard and attempt to reach the limits of your genetic potential. When Arnold started training at fifteen he had no way of knowing what the future held. Genetics aside, it was his unrelenting drive and ambition that helped him achieve so much in the sport of bodybuilding. Almost anything is possible with the right commitment.

Psychological Factors

There are, no doubt, tens of thousands of genetic anomalies who possess the necessary attributes for building large muscles, but there are only hundreds, maybe fewer, who also have the necessary drive and ambition to actualize that potential. Given a cross-section of 100,000 males, there might be twenty who have extraordinary physical potential. Of those twenty, perhaps two will have the determination to undertake the years of hard training necessary to develop an exceptionally muscular physique. This number will always be very small because it requires an almost fanatical commitment to pursue any endeavor to the absolute limit. Most people never exert themselves maximally.

It's important, for those of you seriously pursuing bodybuilding, to form a strong, vivid picture of what you want to look like. This vision of a physical ideal will help you keep your motivation high. You may be able to psyche yourself a little and increase your drive, but the individual must cultivate that germ of ambition that lies within.

The Zen master says, "There is happiness in difficulty, difficulty in happiness. When you do something difficult you should be completely involved in it. You should devote yourself to it completely."

The most amazing aspect of the Mentzer Method is that once you fully understand the basic physiological principles involved, you can adjust the training procedure to meet your individual needs. In essence you can be your own trainer. This is as important for the beginner as for the seasoned bodybuilder. If you're seeking to improve your overall fitness level, you can manipulate the intensity and duration of the exercises to achieve the desired training effect and skeletal-muscle development. On the other hand, the aspiring bodybuilder, whose goal is the acquisition of as much muscle tissue as possible, can tailor the training to meet this goal.

First, however, the beginner and the serious bodybuilder must grasp the details of the method.

No Mystery Involved

Bodybuilders are believers. For decades they've been told each person is different and therefore each has to discover what works for him in building muscle. It's a case of having to continually reinvent the wheel. It's true, of course, that we're all different and unique to some degree, but the differences fall within a rather narrow range.

My pectoral muscles may respond better to bench presses than to flys but that's not necessarily true for everyone. The variation is the result of the difference in anatomical structure. While title holder Tom Platz reduces his calorie intake to 3,000 a day before a contest in order to get more "cut up," I have to reduce my intake to 1,500 to achieve the same result. These differences in anatomy and metabolism notwithstanding, the laws of physiology are the same for the entire species. If this wasn't true, medical science wouldn't exist. What makes medical science work is the fact that data gathered from studies of a relatively small number of individuals can then be applied to the entire human population. It is logical, therefore, that the biochemical changes that result in muscle growth are essentially the same for everyone. The cause of these cellular changes—high-intensity exercise—is also the same for everyone. Intensity in bodybuilding can best be defined as the percentage of momentary effort a person is capable of exerting.

Highly repetitive exercise—bicycling, swimming, distance running—requires very little momentary exertion and therefore doesn't stimulate much muscle growth. This means that the body-builder who wants to increase muscular size must regularly attempt to perform those repetitions that seem impossible at the moment. In attempting that last, seemingly impossible repetition, the body is forced to dip into its reserves and the body has only a limited amount of reserve strength. To protect itself from continued assaults on these precious reserves, the body increases its ability to meet heavy stress. This compensatory development occurs as greater muscle mass and enhanced strength.

Intensity is obviously a relative matter. For the beginner who has never exercised, any demand on the body will represent a dramatic increase in intensity. But the body will immediately begin to adapt to these demands by building more and stronger muscle.

For the beginner or the advanced weight trainer, new growth is stimulated only by a step up the ladder of intensity.

Increasing Intensity

First of all, don't confuse training harder with training longer. Physical activity is not synonymous with physical training. Physical activity has to be maintained at a certain level of intensity before it results in a physical training effect. It follows that as you exert yourself more intensely, you will be using less time for your exertion. Intensity of effort and duration of effort are mutually exclusive.

The level of intensity can be increased in three ways:

1) By increasing the weight being used
2) By decreasing the amount of time taken to perform a certain amount of work
3) By carrying each set to a point of momentary total failure

Weight

As your strength increases, you must increase the amount of weight you're using. Let's say you now press 100 pounds for a maximum of six repetitions. Next week you may be able to do ten repetitions with that weight. At that point you should increase the weight you're using by about 10 percent or a little more, enough to bring your maximum number of repetitions back down to six. If you continue to use the 100 pounds after your strength has increased, you will be performing at a submaximal level and you'll primarily be increasing your endurance, not your strength. This is the nature of progressive weight training. You can increase muscular strength and size only by progressively moving up the intensity gauge.

Time

If your present training routine takes two hours, completing the same amount of work in one hour will double the intensity and effectiveness of the activity. It's a question of simple arithmetic but it must be accomplished gradually and progressively. Decreasing the time doesn't mean just doing your reps faster. In fact, you must continue to perform your exercises slowly and in good form. You pick up the time in other ways.

Often it's only a matter of motivation and concentration. I practically guarantee you can pick up at least twenty minutes by cutting down on the time you spend talking to your friends between sets and by speeding up your weight changes.

The stress increases as you work to decrease your overall training time and, at first, you may need a couple of minutes rest between sets. That's all right. If you race from one exercise to another, it may make you light-headed or nauseous, but it will certainly reduce your training efficiency and the intensity of effort required to stimulate muscular growth. As I've said all along, take it easy and your progress will be steady.

Momentary Total Failure

The third method of increasing the level of intensity is training to a point of total failure, a vague term that needs some explaining. Total failure doesn't mean continuing a set until you can't perform even a partial movement. It doesn't mean a set is finished when a complete repetition is no longer possible. It doesn't refer to the duration of training sessions. Nor does it mean that you should do set after endless set until you're so exhausted you have to end the workout. It means something else entirely.

The skeletal muscles have three levels of strength. The first level, and the weakest, is the ability of the muscle to raise a weight from a position of full extension to one of full contraction (as in a curl). This is also called positive strength or concentric contraction. The muscle is stronger in a position of stasis (or balance), the second level of strength, than in contraction. This means you can hold more weight at any given point in a muscle's range of motion than the muscle can raise in a positive contraction. If you can curl a maximum weight of 125 pounds for one repetition, then you can hold 150 pounds or more for several seconds at any point in the range of motion of the curl.

The third level of strength, the strongest, is the ability of the muscle to lower a weight under control from a fully contracted to a fully extended position. This lengthening of the muscle as it lowers a weight is known as negative or eccentric exercise. If you are capable of curling 125 pounds for one repetition and holding 150 pounds in a static position at any point in that curl, then you can lower 175–200 pounds in a curl. Remember that maximal tension is produced when the muscle lengthens and it declines as the muscle shortens. Of course, you're effectively limited by your positive strength since, if you can't lift a weight, you can't possibly perform the negative work of lowering it.

What is meant, then, by total muscular failure is a state where you have exhausted all three levels of muscular strength.

For example, if you press 150 pounds for a maximum of ten repetitions, you may have exhausted your positive strength but you're only one third of the way to total failure since you still have a generous measure of static- and negative-level strength available. It's therefore also clear that you haven't trained with maximum intensity since you haven't exerted 100 percent of your momentary ability. And this can only be accomplished if you continue after the last positive repetition to somehow lower the weight under control to a point of failure (and you can't do that without help). Then, and only then, will you have reached a point of *total* muscular failure and exerted maximum intensity of effort as well.

The fact that many bodybuilders have built outstanding physiques with low-intensity, marathon workouts of three hours a day, six days a week, proves nothing. I maintain, as do exercise physiologists, that these people would have developed farther and faster if they had used the Mentzer Method of training. Anyone, and I mean anyone, who trains six days a week, four hours a day, and then says he trains hard, doesn't have any idea what hard training really is. He may be training diligently, and he may be training for a long time, but he isn't training hard. High-intensity training is brutally hard and until you experience it for yourself or watch someone else, you can't possibly appreciate the effort involved.

The Advanced Bodybuilder

If you've been training at least a year or more you're probably pretty frustrated because your progress has slowed way down. Those exhilarating gains during the early months of training are by now being measured in millimeters rather than inches. This slowdown is caused by the body's adaptation to the level of intensity of your workout. Any further progress will necessitate greater effort. There are a couple of techniques available that will increase training intensity, help you off that plateau, and put you back on the road to greater progress.

Pre-Exhaustion

To review for a moment. Muscle growth is stimulated by intense exercise. Maximum progress can only be achieved by maximum exertion, that is, 100 percent of your momentary ability must be expended on every single exercise.

This isn't always possible in many conventional exercises because of muscular "weak links." When doing inclined presses, for example, the work of the pectoral muscles is limited because of the involvement of the smaller and weaker triceps. The point of failure in the inclined press will be reached when the triceps (the weak links) fail. This is long before the bigger and stronger pectorals are exhausted. A similar problem exists when the latissimus dorsi muscles are worked with such conventional exercises as rows, chins, or pull-downs on the lat machine. The biceps (the weak links), worked along with the lats in these exercises, fail before the lats become fatigued. But you can work around these weak links by using an isolation exercise for the stronger muscles before performing the compound exercise. Dumbbell flys, cable crossovers, or Nautilus chest are ideal isolation exercises for the pecs, and when carried to total failure will "pre-exhaust" the pecs while preserving the strength of the triceps.

This isolation exercise must be followed *immediately* with absolutely no rest by a compound exercise—dips or incline presses—that allows the fresh triceps to serve the exhausted pecs. The triceps now have a temporary strength advantage over the pecs and this forces the pecs to continue to contract closer to 100 percent of their momentary strength. If you delay as little as three seconds in moving from the isolation to the compound exercise, the primary muscle group (in this case the pecs) will regain up to 50 percent of its original strength, thus making the auxiliary muscle the weak link again. When the isolation-compound cycle has been completed, it's all right to rest for as long as necessary before moving ahead in your workout.

Forced Repetitions

While pre-exhaustion is a significant new concept in bodybuilding technique, forced repetitions, another method of raising intensity, are an idea that has been around for years. When using forced repetitions, choose a weight for each exercise that will allow six strict reps and through sheer will and determination two or three more. When you've completed as many strict positive reps as possible, have a training partner help you complete the remaining two or three forced reps. This help should be just enough to make the last reps possible. The effort on your part should be fierce. It may take as long as six seconds just to raise the weight. The idea is to increase the intensity by forcing you to exert more of your momentary ability.

At this point you're two thirds of the way to exhaustion. But you'll still have strength enough to perform the negative action of lowering the weight.

Negative Resistance

Even after the exertion of the forced reps your negative strength is still available and until you've exhausted this last and greatest level of strength, you can't truly say that you've trained to the point of total failure.

Move directly from the forced reps to the negative reps by having your partner raise the weight to the top position for the exercise. Your job now is to lower the weight, keeping it under control. The first few negatives will seem relatively easy and you'll be able to lower the weight slowly. It's even possible to stop the downward motion of the weight during the first few negatives because some of your static strength will still be available. Then it gets tougher. The downward speed of the weight will increase and you won't have as much control. At this point your static strength will be gone and after another two or three reps you'll be forced to stop because you won't be able to control the weight. Stop before the weight gets out of control because it's dangerous to have a weight yank a muscle out of the contracted position.

You will now have trained the muscle group involved to total failure. I know this is a rather long description, but part of the Mentzer Method is a complete understanding of the principles involved, and exercising to total failure is one of my basic principles. To repeat: these exercises—as is obvious by now—are only for the serious, dedicated bodybuilder who has completely mastered the three-sequence weight-training program.

Rest-Pause Training

When increases in muscular size and strength seemingly come to a halt even though you've continued to train faithfully, you'll know that your body has fully adapted to a certain level of training intensity. This, as I said before, necessitates a further step up the ladder of intensity.

For a while, adding weight and decreasing training time will be enough to up your training effort the notches required to stimulate muscular growth. The truly advanced bodybuilder who has been training for years and has developed considerable size and strength will have reached a level of fitness where further change is limited by a complex of physiological barriers.

As the muscles grow bigger and stronger, major muscular contractions exert greater demands on the body's resources. More oxygen and more fuel in the form of glucose are demanded and the greater build-up of waste products needs to be eliminated. It's obvious that a twenty-inch arm contracting with maximum force and intensity places a much higher demand on the body's resources than a twelve-inch arm contracting maximally.

This point was brought home to me with great clarity during an experience I had while sharing a training session with an aspiring teenage bodybuilder I occasionally work out with.

I was doing a set of concentration curls with an eighty-pound dumbbell and my young partner was doing the same exercise with a twenty-five-pound dumbbell. When I finished my set I was sweating buckets and breathing like a race horse while my friend was breathing almost normally and seemed fresh as a daisy. He was very happy to point this fact out to me and frankly I was puzzled. After thinking about it though, I realized that while he seemed to be exerting himself as much as I was, in actuality, I was working much harder and exerting more force because of my body size and, as a result, was stressing myself much more than he was.

This led me to rest-pause training. I reached an impasse in my development last year. I discovered that my strength and my increased ability to exert myself proved so taxing that oxygen debt and waste build-up was immediate. It began with the first repetition of a six-repetition set and prevented maximum contraction throughout the set. What was needed was an ultra-intense method of training that somehow circumvented the oxygen-debt and waste-buildup problem that was preventing a maximum effort.

I was able to do this by using a long-forgotten but highly productive training method known as "rest-pause." Rest-pause requires that you thoroughly warm up the particular muscle involved in the exercise and then perform the exercise with a weight that requires a maximum effort to complete one repetition. When the one maximum rep is completed, the weight is put down. After about a ten-second rest, a second repetition is performed with the same weight (or slightly lighter if necessary). This routine is repeated four times. Each rep must be an all-out effort using perfectly strict form and paying special attention to the lowering (or negative) movement of the weight. I find that with most exercises a slight decrease in weight is necessary after each repetition.

Rest-pause is very taxing so don't try to do more than one set for each exercise or more than three exercises per muscle. Remember, when training intensity increases, there must be a corresponding decrease in duration of training time.

Since rest-pause requires a quantum leap in intensity, the cutback in training time is dramatic. During some workouts I perform as few as seven total sets, and never more than thirteen, while working the entire body from legs to arms. At most I'll use rest-pause training only twice a week.

This is a very severe form of exercise and I advise it only for the most advanced bodybuilders, those people who have spent years working themselves to the top rung of the intensity ladder.

Training Partner

As you progress and become more serious about your training, a training partner can become an important element in your continued progress. It's crucial that your partner be personally compatible, that you share the same enthusiasm for training, and that your strength is comparable, the better to push each other during workouts.

In the more advanced training techniques involving forced and negative repetitions, a training partner is all but indispensable. As you move through intense sets toward a point of failure your partner can provide physical assistance for those final, nearly impossible, reps.

A partner is a psychological plus as well. Knowing your friend is waiting for you at the gym will force you to train even on those days when you'd rather do almost anything else. And the verbal encouragement you give each other during a workout can produce much higher levels of performance.

If you choose to work without a partner, some of the exercises that follow will be more difficult. You'll have to innovate, to vary a bit. For example, forced reps become more difficult. Take behind-the-neck presses. At the point in a set where you can no longer complete a full rep, you'll have to bend your knees slightly and heave to get the weight moving and be able to finish alone. You can do the dips by standing up on a chair to reach the top position for the negatives. It's harder but still possible, of course.

Just remember, whether you train with a partner or by yourself, the important thing is that you train as hard as possible.

Mental Attitude

As I've said earlier, all the natural ability in the world is worthless without the motivation to put it to use. Even physiologists, who place such great stock in genetic endowment, recognize that given a high level of ability, motivation can be *the* most important factor in success.

Through the years I've learned that I train with 100 percent effort, at the outer limits, only in the final weeks of preparation for a contest. Knowing I'll soon be on stage with the world's greatest bodybuilders, engaged in a physical and mental competition in front of thousands of cheering people, is the spark that fans the flames of pride and desire deep within me. At these times I think of the gym as a battlefield. The barbells are my enemies, the resistance I must overcome. My strength seems to skyrocket. My training poundages are awesome—200 pounds for some curls, 400 pounds for inclined presses, 1,000 pounds for leg presses. At times my training effort is so inspired, so fierce, the battle so all consuming, that the whole gym will stop and watch.

Top athletes in all sports must subject themselves to years of arduous training, must be willing to endure the long hours of ultimate effort necessary to attain their specific goals.

The greatest resistance encountered on the road to great athletic achievement is not the body, however, it's the mind. It's not the weights, the hours, the weather, the equipment, it's the mind. The well-trained body is capable of near-maximum effort at any time. Any type of activity, mental or physical, places certain demands on the body's resources. As the effort required for a particular activity increases, so does the demand on our bodies. What usually gives out first is the mind, not the body.

For the serious bodybuilder engaged in high-intensity exercise on a regular basis, the mind becomes an obstacle that must be overcome almost daily. The mind is clever. It enables us to think of very plausible excuses. Psychosomatic problems—tiredness, headache, nausea, and anxiety—stand in the way much more often than strains, pulls, soreness, or real fatigue. Only a strong mind possessed of a vivid orienting vision can overcome these obstacles. A clear image of the body you *want* to develop can motivate you to train. Arnold Schwarzenegger, in his mind's eye, saw his biceps as big mountains while he was doing his curls. You, too, must learn to visualize yourself growing to meet your ideal. Before each workout, take the time to close your eyes and concentrate on a movielike image of yourself going through your entire workout, breaking records in weight and training intensity. Go to the gym hyped up, in a state of high physical and emotional tension, seething with a desire to battle the weights. And to win.

As your muscles grow, as your strength increases, you'll feel an enhancement of life and power, a new motivation. This physical and mental growth will continue to serve as an expression of your victorious will.

How Much and How Often

I recommend a four-day-a-week program for the serious bodybuilder who wants to follow the program outlined later in this chapter. This is definitely flexible—it may be too much for some—but don't try more than four days even if you're not having any problems. If you find you're getting fatigued and having trouble recuperating from the high-intensity effort, by all means cut back.

If you're doing two cycles for each body part, cut back to one. If you're training two days and resting one, you can rest a day after each workout.

I don't advise including negative repetitions at the end of each and every exercise every workout because they increase the intensity of the work dramatically. Just try to perform negatives for each body part once a week. It's not necessary to do the whole body in the same workout.

If you train the whole body in one day, work the largest muscles first and then follow a descending order to the smallest. This means move from the legs to the back, the chest, the deltoids, and then the arms.

I'm not kidding when I say high-intensity training is brutal. Don't hurry through the workout at first. Give your body plenty of time to adapt to the higher stress before speeding up your pace. It may take as long as an hour and a half to complete the routines at first but your time will gradually decrease until it takes only thirty minutes. It's imperative to reduce the workout time because intensity, as I've said, is directly related to the time it takes to complete a given amount of work.

Here's a final reminder: Training every day is a serious mistake. It won't speed up your development in size or strength. Following a workout, the body must have time to recover the energy it has expended. When too much energy is spent during training (six days a week, twenty sets for each body part) the body has difficulty merely regenerating used resources. There is nothing left for growth.

Remember it takes years to build a title-winning physique. Try to be patient.

The Workout

The following routines are designed for a four-day-a-week workout schedule. Vary this as you see fit and as your body dictates but be sure to do all the suggested exercises in the order they are given. This will assure a complete workout for the entire body.

Most of these exercises have been described in the previous chapters. A few haven't been discussed, but if you're a serious bodybuilder you'll already know the techniques involved. For that reason I'm not going into detail here. I don't think you'll have any problems.

Monday and Thursday

Legs: 1) Leg extensions ⎫
                   ⎬ One cycle *
        2) Leg presses ⎭
        3) Squats—one set
        4) Leg curls—one set
        5) Toe raises—two or three sets

Alternate isolation exercise—The leg extension is the only exercise that effectively isolates the frontal thigh muscles. If a leg curl machine isn't available, hyperextensions or stiff-legged dead lifts will do as substitutions.

Alternate compound exercises—Perform cycles of squats immediately after the leg extension if there is no leg-press machine available.

Note: Squats involve much heavier weights and can cause damage to the lower back if you're not very careful. For that reason I suggest that you use a weight that allows for approximately ten reps and that you stop at the point of positive failure rather than go on to total failure with negative reps.

Chest: 1) Dumbbell flys ⎫
                         ⎬ Two cycles
        2) Incline presses with barbell or ⎪
           dumbbells ⎭

Alternate isolation exercises—French presses, cable extensions, Nautilus tricep extensions, and barbell extensions are good isolation exercises.

Alternate compound exercises—Close-grip barbell benchpresses or bench dips.

---

* Cycle means the two exercises are to be done in rapid succession with absolutely no rest. In this case, leg extensions followed by leg presses.

Tuesday and Friday

Lats:
1) Stiff-arm pull-down on lat machine
2) Close-grip, palms-up pull-down
} Two cycles
3) One-arm dumbbell row— two sets

Alternate isolation exercises—Nautilus pull-over, Nautilus behind-neck torso, and pull-overs across bench with either barbell or dumbbells.

Alternate compound exercises—Barbell rows, cable rows, and close-grip palms-up chins.

Trapezius:
1) Shrugs
2) Upright rows
} Two cycles

Alternate isolation exercises—Shrugs can be performed with a barbell, dumbbells, or on the Nautilis multi-exercise machine.

Alternate compound exercise—High pulls with barbell, barbell cleans, and dead-hang snatches.

Deltoids:
1) Dumbbell laterals
2) Press behind neck
} Two cycles
3) Bent-over dumbbell laterals—two sets

Alternate isolation exercise—Nautilus shoulder.

Alternate compound exercises—Dumbbell presses with elbows pointed to the sides and the Nautilus press unit.

Biceps:
1) Barbell curls
2) Palms-up chins
} Two cycles

Alternate isolation exercises—Any type of curl.

Alternate compound exercise—Palms-up pull-down on lat machine.

Points to Remember

• There should be no rest time between the first and second exercises of a cycle.

• Work to cut down your total exercise time but don't rush so much that you compromise your workout efficiency.

• All movements should be slow and deliberate with no sudden jerks to get the weight moving.

• Complete the full range of motion (from full extension to full contraction and back again) in a deliberate style.

• Progressively increase your weights as you gain strength but don't sacrifice proper technique. As a rule of thumb increase the weight by 10 percent when the weight that allowed six repetitions allows nine.

• Fight the tendency to add more sets to these workouts. Doing more is rarely the answer to stimulating growth—harder is the answer. And the harder you train, the shorter the time you'll be physically able to train.

• Don't think you can make up for performing sets haphazardly by doing more haphazard sets.

• Change the exercises whenever you want, every workout if you feel like it. The important thing is that you stick to the underlying principles.

• Don't include the forced reps, negative resistance, or rest-pause sequences for every body part every workout. Working each body part to total failure once a week is sufficient.

• Never, never train more than four days a week. In most cases three days a week is enough. Enough time must be allowed between workouts for recovery and growth.

• This workout is not a guarantee of a Mr. America physique. No workout plan can guarantee anything. It will allow you to gain only as rapidly as dictated by the limits of your genetic potential.

The Bodybuilder and Nutrition

Bodybuilders have always placed a great deal of emphasis on nutrition, and rightly so. Proper nutrition is important to physical performance and it is vital to the development of a great physique.

But there is a vast difference between nutrition and proper nutrition. Merely gorging yourself with excessive quantities of protein and vitamins is not proper nutrition. The same mistaken notion that has led bodybuilders to believe marathon training is good has been applied to dieting as well: If 100 grams of protein a day is recommended for your body weight, then 300 grams must be three times as effective. Note this fact: It has yet to be proven that more than enough of an essential element of nutrition is better than just enough.

The human body has specific daily needs for all the important nutrients but that need is relatively small. Forcing down huge quantities of these elements won't induce your body to utilize more than it needs and certainly won't promote faster muscular growth. The most important factor in nutrition for those seeking to build muscle, and everyone else for that matter, is a well-balanced diet. In all probability, this diet will provide your daily nutritional needs and prevent you from taking in so many calories that you get fat in the process. The well-balanced diet must include all the basic nutrients needed to keep the body functioning properly. This means fairly sizable quantities of the macronutrients—protein, fats, carbohydrates, and water—and much smaller quantities of the micronutrients—vitamins and minerals. (See Part I, Chapter 6.)

Water—Believe it or not, water is one of the most important nutrients for building muscle tissue. Most bodybuilders equate muscle with protein but muscle tissue is 70 percent water and only 20 percent protein. Why then has protein been billed as *the* most essential nutrient for building muscle? Because the so-called health-food purveyors can't sell water through the mail like protein products. You can get as much good water as you need from the kitchen faucet and it's almost free. This doesn't mean that you should start gulping five gallons of water a day to build muscle faster. Just let your natural desire for liquids govern your intake. Excess beyond need will result only in more trips to the bathroom.

Protein—Yes, protein is important for building muscles. It is the body's most important building material. In fact, protein in Greek means "of first importance." It does not mean "of only importance," however. Protein is required for growth, maintenance, and repair of muscle tissue and the body in general.

Protein requirements depend almost entirely on your body weight, not your level of physical activity, because it is not used as fuel as long as the body's energy supply is adequate. The rule of thumb is one gram of protein per day for every two pounds of body weight. There is no reason to buy expensive supplements since this amount of protein can be obtained from any well-balanced diet that includes meat, fish, or dairy products. I maintain my weight at about 220 pounds and consume about 60 grams of protein a day, less than recommended for my weight, and I'm still growing muscle.

As I said before, muscle growth is a very slow process. On a daily basis it really can't be detected at all. A ten-pound gain in a year would amount to less than half an ounce a day.

How much protein beyond maintenance requirements would you need to gain a half ounce of muscle a day? Approximately 1 gram, the amount in one ounce of whole milk, an eighth of an ounce of tuna, or a half slice of bacon. You can even get that 1 gram from a single carrot. Yet this extra protein would be enough to build ten pounds of muscle a year.

Think about that the next time you make an investment in a can of protein supplement.

Carbohydrates—If protein has been the most overemphasized nutrient, then carbohydrates have been the most maligned. Food faddists and even some nutritionists blame carbohydrates for everything from heart disease and depression to dandruff.

The fact is that the human body, especially the brain and nervous system, lives almost entirely on glucose, the chemically processed form in which carbohydrates are finally utilized by the body. The choice of fuel for the working muscle is limited to carbohydrate and fat, primarily carbohydrate. You can't build muscle without carbohydrates for two reasons. First, without adequate sugar in your system you won't be able to train with the intensity and energy necessary to build muscle through dynamic exercise, and second, each gram of glucose (taken from carbohydrates) stores three grams of water, the primary element in muscle tissues.

Try to obtain most of your carbohydrates from unrefined or natural foods (not necessarily health foods) such as fruit, grains, and vegetables. The sugar in refined foods—candy, cake, ice cream—is ultimately the same as far as the body is concerned since all sugar ends up as glucose by the time it enters the bloodstream, but these foods are deficient in vitamins and minerals and are high in fat and calories. They should be kept to a minimum.

Fats—A certain amount of fat is important to a well-balanced diet. Fat provides fuel, especially at high levels of physical activity, and fat is calorie dense, providing nine calories per gram compared to four calories per gram for carbohydrates and proteins. Low-fat diets may help you lose weight but you'll be cutting out an important fuel source and potentially reducing your energy level. On the other hand, elevated fat levels in the blood can be a risk. There is evidence that the intake of fatty substances can be a factor in the development of atherosclerosis.

Vitamins and Minerals—These micronutrients (so called because the body needs such small quantities on a daily basis) combine with some of the body's enzymes and act as biochemical catalysts to utilize the macronutrients. Minerals are especially important to the bodybuilder because they act as electrolytes which aid in maintaining water balance, regulating temperature, and controlling muscular activity. If you're eating a well-balanced diet, you're getting all the vitamins and minerals you need. If, for whatever reason, it's not always possible to eat well, a multiple vitamin and mineral supplement may be useful. Remember micro means small. The body needs less than ⅛ of a teaspoon of vitamins and minerals a day.

Balancing Calories

Food supplies calories, which are converted to energy. If you're getting enough protein but not enough calories, the body will eventually convert the protein to glucose and use it for fuel. Carbohydrates and fats are the body's preferred fuel and this allows protein to do its job of growth and maintenance. Most nutritionists recommend that the daily allotment of calories should consist of at least 50 percent carbohydrates, no more than 35 percent fats, and about 15 percent proteins. If your daily maintenance need is 3,000 calories, then approximately 1,500 should be carbohydrates, 1,050 fats, and 450 proteins.

Earlier in this book (see Part I Chapter 6) I described how to determine your BMR. If you are high strung with a high metabolic rate, then you'll burn more calories than the average person just maintaining life. This means you'll have to eat more to maintain yourself and even more to grow. If this is your problem, try to eat calorie-dense food (fats) which will help keep the volume of your consumption down and prevent bloating and digestion problems.

After determining your maintenance needs by following the formula, you'll be able to adjust your calorie intake as you train harder to stimulate muscular growth. A few calories a day, no more than 200 above maintenance, will provide for that growth.

Anyone can gain weight by merely eating more calories than are expended. But just overeating will do nothing but make you fat, and fat serves no purpose for the bodybuilder.

Chapter 6

Age Is a State of Mind

I will never forget the 1977 Mr. Olympia contest. It was an exciting event from beginning to end, but the most electrifying moment for me came during the final judging when Ed Corney, who won the Mr. Universe title back in 1972, took the posing platform. What followed was the most sensational posing performance I've ever seen. Ed brought down the house and received one of the greatest ovations in bodybuilding history in the process. Ed Corney was forty-four years old at the time. He looked twenty-four and performed with the vigor and enthusiasm of a teenager. He's still competing today and he's very tough to beat.

Ed Corney is just one example of the truth in the old saying, "Life begins at forty." Other bodybuilders—Bill Pearl, John Grimek, Larry Scott—now in their forties, fifties, and sixties are still in top shape and capable of competing. And there are currently an impressive number of "older" professional athletes in baseball, football, track and field, tennis, and hockey who, as they approach forty, are still competing and excelling. It's not only professionals though. The newspapers and magazines are full of stories of older amateur athletes who seem to be possessed of inexhaustible supplies of energy. An octogenarian conducts an exercise program at a New York City YMCA, seventy-year-olds regularly run in the Boston Marathon, and the seniors brackets in tennis tournaments all over the country are filled. None of these people are genetic freaks but every one of them will tell you there is no substitute for physical and mental fitness and that they keep up with the "kids" by training and watching their weight all year round. Interestingly, most of these people have always been fit and regular exercise has been an important element in their lives. And a surprising number of older, well-conditioned people, especially men, have been weight trainers at one time in their lives. Many of them still are.

I firmly believe you're only as old as you feel. Age is more a state of mind than a matter of chronology, if you're healthy. Vitality, stamina, and virility—the keys to the quality of your life at any age—depend largely on the state of your physical and mental health. And good health depends on a combination of exercise and a balanced diet.

People must remain physically active or they deteriorate. C. Carson Conrad, executive director of the President's Council on Physical Fitness and Sports, says it plainly: "If you just sit around, you can watch bones and muscles atrophy. If you sit around and wait to die, you won't have long to wait."

Aging, of course, is a process we can't stop. Physiological maturity and maximum strength are reached in our early twenties. At around twenty-five or so, most people reach their "prime." Athletic ability also reaches its peak in the mid-twenties. Ironically, at almost exactly that point of maximum strength, endurance, and all-around ability, the slow but steady process of the body's deterioration begins.

And though nothing can be done about this decline it is possible to control the physical and mental changes that accompany the chronological inexorability of age. That measure of control is achieved by maintaining a high level of physical fitness.

As people grow older they generally become less physically active. At the same time they begin to eat more and are less careful about eating a balanced diet. They put on weight and become less active still. It's a vicious circle. Muscles shrink from disuse and are replaced by fat. Strength decreases gradually. The strength of a sixty-five-year-old is approximately 80 percent of what it was when the person was twenty-five. Bones become less dense and suffer from disuse just as muscles do. The heart's ability to eject blood into the main artery (stroke volume) decreases and there is a decline in the maximum heart rate. Blood pressure goes up and maximum aerobic power declines. At 50 percent maximum aerobic power the heart rate of a twenty-five-year-old man is about 130, but with the same relative work load the heart rate of a sixty-five-year-old is 110. During exercise the arterial blood pressure is higher in the old than in the young. Nerve signals lose speed in transmission. The size of the brain decreases and the body's defenses against disease and stress diminish. The ability to taste and smell degenerates, hair turns gray or falls out, and the sight begins to weaken.

It's some dreary picture. But before you cash in your chips and leave the game early, remember that the variation between individuals is great. While a group of ten-year-olds won't vary much from child to child, a group of fifty- or sixty-year-olds will show tremendous differences. Two sixty-year-olds can be as different as life and death. One can be vigorous, virile, trim, straight, and vital in every way and the other can be fat, hobbling, inactive, and very old in appearance. It's this variation that must be kept in mind. It's possible to fight the effects of aging, and to win.

It doesn't matter when you start a physical fitness program, only that you do get started. What more motivation do you need than the chance to avoid many of the depressing effects of age just listed, or the warning that, "If you sit around and wait to die, you won't have long to wait"?

Here are some encouraging words from the physiologists. A 1976 study of men fifty-five to seventy who had been physically inactive for a minimum of twenty years, showed that after eight weeks of training, the average increase in the group's maximum oxygen intake—the measure of aerobic power—was twenty percent. This happened in only eight weeks and occurred after twenty years of sedentary existence. This is a very encouraging finding. Similar results were reported in another study of thirty-nine to sixty-year-olds. An experiment involving the middle-aged staff of a midwestern university corroborated these positive conclusions. It seems apparent from these studies that the "normal" decline in maximum oxygen intake that occurs after age twenty can be modified by regular training and can result in the rejuvenation of fifteen to twenty years in this particular measure of fitness. Other research has shown that muscular exercise helps preserve bone strength. And while it is true that older people are less trainable than younger people, the effects of exercise training can be noticed even in the very old.

If you have maintained a reasonable level of fitness most of your life, you will have fewer problems in retaining or improving that state of fitness. Studies of highly trained athletes have shown that their maximum heart rate and maximum aerobic power remain higher than average even fifteen years after regular training ends. If training is started again, that higher-than-average figure can be raised even more, though it probably will never reach its former level.

If you're forty or more, here are some points to keep in mind about exercise.

Medical Examination

If you've been inactive or only moderately active for several years, I strongly advise you to see a doctor before beginning this, or any, exercise program. It's vital that you know your general state of health and specifically that you know your maximum heart rate. If you have had any heart problems at all, you must see a doctor—especially when contemplating a weight-training program. As I said earlier, blood pressure and heart rate are higher in arm work than in leg work. This results in a heavy load for the heart. People with heart disease, or completely untrained older people, may find weight training hazardous because of the amount of arm work involved. Even carrying groceries can be dangerous for cardiac patients. Running, on the other hand, involves very little arm work and can be a useful conditioner under controlled circumstances.

Injuries

The fitness boom has created a tremendous amount of new business for doctors. Not only are they seeing more patients for physical checkups, they are also seeing more older people and previously sedentary people who have suffered some sort of injury. A good deal of flexibility and muscular strength is lost through the years, even when you remain active, and as you grow older you are more susceptible to injury. Knees, ankles, and other joints are especially delicate. Muscles, ligaments, and tendons are more easily pulled and strained. Fractures are not uncommon. This simply means you should begin your training gradually, testing the body as you go, listening to it, and accepting its limitations.

Pulse

Be aware of your pulse rate and the age-adjusted level you determined as your training target. Even exercise at 50 percent of maximum, if sustained for several minutes, can be beneficial for the cardiovascular system. Take your pulse as often as you think it's necessary and stop working out immediately if you detect an irregular or a higher-than-normal rate.

Diet

You have already determined your BMR and your total calorie needs for body maintenance (BMR plus activity level). The body's balance is remarkably delicate so it's very important to control energy intake as you get older. Continue to adjust your BMR 2 percent for every decade of age and stick with the new figure. Even a slight drop in your activity level, perfectly normal with age, coupled with the same rate of calorie intake, can result in weight gain. A few hundred calories a day will add up to a pound in a very few days.

Try to maintain a well-balanced diet as well. Pay particular attention to the amount of fat, sugar, and salt in your diet and try to eat more vegetables. Those few extra pounds, difficult to lose at any age, are even harder to lose as you get older.

The Mentzer Method

If you've been training or have kept yourself in decent shape most of your life, there is no reason why you can't undertake the complete exercise program I recommend. One of the beauties of the Mentzer Method is that it is easily controllable. The frequency, duration, and intensity of your workouts are completely under your control. You can monitor your pulse at any time. Just start gradually and work yourself up to the level of fitness that satisfies you.

For those who are older and have been sedentary for some time, I suggest the modified program detailed in the chapter on breaking in. Stick with that program for six months, then if you judge yourself ready to move up the ladder of intensity, do it gradually.

A Final Note

People often ask me if any form of exercise is better than no exercise at all. My answer is an emphatic no. The major reason for the physical decline experienced with age is the decrease in the body's ability to transport oxygen—cardiovascular fitness. The only way to increase this ability is through vigorous exercise that produces a cardiovascular training effect. Such vigorous exercise can actually reverse the body's downward slide and will slow further decline. Bowling, golf, and softball provide about as much exercise as driving your car, which is to say no exercise at all. For the type of fitness I'm talking about, intense physical activity is an absolute requirement. You have to break a sweat.

Regular, intense exercise is the only way to stay young and maintain a high level of fitness and well-being. Methuselah, the biblical patriarch, is said to have lived more than 900 years. It wouldn't surprise me at all to learn that he spent three or four hundred years as a weight trainer. I know of no other physical fitness activity that could have kept him in such good condition for so long.

Index